Contemporary Approach to Trauma and Emergency Surgery

Edited by Ozgur Karcioglu and Canan Akman

Published in London, United Kingdom

Contemporary Approach to Trauma and Emergency Surgery
http://dx.doi.org/10.5772/intechopen.1001692
Edited by Ozgur Karcioglu and Canan Akman

Contributors
Alberto De La Espriella, Amalia Angélica Reyes Pérez, Brenda Lizbeth González Zúñiga, Canan Akman, Davide Luppi, Erdal Güngör, Fabrizio Giuseppe Bonanno, Gabriela María Mora Martínez, Gustavo Adrián Soto Hernandez, Helen Yu, Maurizio Zizzo, Ozgur Karcioglu, Ramón Ulises Soberano Burguete, Rodolfo Antonio Valerio Aguirre, Ruggero Bollino, Theno Alexandro Turrubiates Hernández

First published in London, United Kingdom, 2024 by IntechOpen
IntechOpen is the global imprint of INTECHOPEN LIMITED, registered in England and Wales, registration number: 11086078, 167-169 Great Portland Street, London, W1W 5PF, United Kingdom

British Library Cataloguing-in-Publication Data
A catalogue record for this book is available from the British Library

Additional hard and PDF copies can be obtained from orders@intechopen.com

Contemporary Approach to Trauma and Emergency Surgery
Edited by Ozgur Karcioglu and Canan Akman
p. cm.
Print ISBN 978-0-85466-338-5
Online ISBN 978-0-85466-337-8
eBook (PDF) ISBN 978-0-85466-339-2

For EU product safety concerns:
IN TECH d.o.o., Prolaz Marije Krucifikse Kozulić 3, 51000 Rijeka, Croatia,
info@intechopen.com or visit our website at intechopen.com.

Meet the editors

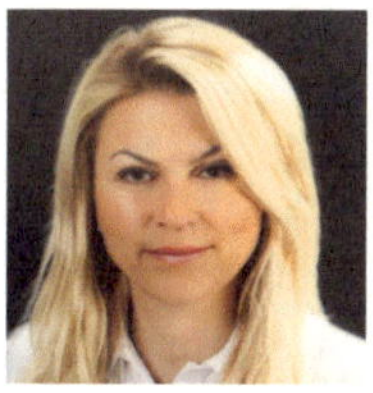

Canan Akman, MD, completed her specialization in emergency medicine at the Department of Emergency Medicine, Hacettepe University, Turkey, in 2011. She is an associate professor in the Faculty of Medicine, Çanakkale Onsekiz Mart University, Turkey. She has published fifty-one articles and nine book chapters to date.

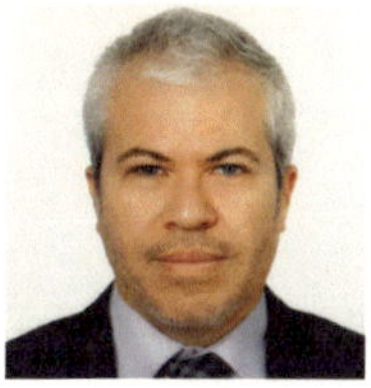

Dr. Ozgur Karcioglu, MD, completed his medical residency at the Department of Emergency Medicine, Dokuz Eylul University, Turkey, in 1998. He completed an International Emergency Medicine Fellowship at Penn State University, USA, in 2005. He is currently the chair of the Department of Emergency Medicine, Taksim Education and Research Hospital, Turkey. He is a founder and board member of the Emergency Medical Association of Turkey. Dr. Karcioglu has published more than 170 articles in scientific journals and five books. He is an instructor of the Advanced Cardiac Life Support Course. His research interests include resuscitation, advanced life support, pain management, airway emergencies, geriatric emergency medicine, disaster medicine, trauma, toxicology, and COVID-19.

Contents

Preface

In the modern era, we have witnessed a significant increase in trauma cases worldwide, and there is the possibility that the number of cases will continue to increase. Especially in developing countries, this frightening situation is mainly attributed to terrorist incidents, warfare, and disaster-like situations including earthquakes and transportation accidents, recreational injuries, and mass casualties. Management and interventions need to be both expedient and accurate in order to accomplish a primary survey of patients and effectively control life-threatening injuries. In a trauma case, the emergency physician should try to rule out the most severe or life-threatening injuries first.

The primary survey involves assessing the patient's airway, breathing, circulation, disability, and exposure/environmental control. This "ABCDE" evaluation includes ensuring airway patency with stabilization of the cervical spine, providing ventilation support (with 5 lt/min O2), ensuring the efficiency of circulation with bleeding control, checking the patient's neurological status (presence of neurological deficit), and ensuring that the patient's clothes are removed during examination. Keeping the patient warm, avoiding hypothermia, insertion of the necessary devices such as nasogastric and urinary catheters, and performing digital rectal examination are important interventions in the management of the severely injured.

Physician evaluations are key to trauma management in establishing a differential diagnosis list, which must be narrowed down to recognize injuries and treat and stabilize patients who have sustained traumatic injuries.

Medical and surgical specialty organizations involved in trauma management come together to establish guidelines on appropriate patient management and selection criteria for those who will benefit from contemporary approaches such as angioembolization, extracorporeal techniques, and resuscitative endovascular balloon occlusion (REBOA) to improve clinical outcomes.

Evaluation of the patient with pelvic injuries and orthopedic cases in the ED mirrors the evaluation of any other patient. The complexity of the approach to these cases by performing many procedures at the same time has brought to the fore the necessity of a team approach in trauma. Most of the time, treatment interventions must be initiated in the ED before a definitive diagnosis is established. The priority order of patients should be re-evaluated at the pre-hospital scene, during patient transport, and upon hospital admission.

Approaches developed for the management of trauma must be flexible to include different subgroups, such as infants, children, pregnant women, the elderly, patients with disabilities, and those with significant comorbidities known before the traumatic injury. For example, thanks to the development of noninvasive monitoring methods and imaging methods such as bedside ultrasonography (POCUS), surgical interventions have become much less commonly employed for a wide range of pediatric solid organ injuries in recent years. Advanced monitoring and imaging techniques such as whole-body computed tomography (PanCT) are on the cusp of practical usage even at the bedside.

Successful management of multiple trauma and related injuries is based on the collaboration of emergency medicine, all other surgical disciplines, intensive care medicine, and almost all disciplines operating in the hospital to achieve and maintain homeostasis, which is the main theme of the book, for positive clinical results.

Hypocrates stated, "Leave the cutting of the stone to the master," which can be translated into current clinical practice as "you shall leave the immediate treatment of the multiple trauma victims to the appropriate team." Appropriate experience can help avoid major pitfalls in trauma care and help provide optimal care for this high-risk group.

Ozgur Karcioglu M.D.
Professor,
Department of Emergency Medicine,
Taksim Education and Research Hospital,
University of Health Sciences,
Fatih, Istanbul, Turkey

Canan Akman M.D.
Associate Professor,
Faculty of Medicine,
Department of Emergency Medicine,
Çanakkale Onsekiz Mart University,
Canakkale, Turkey

Chapter 1

Introductory Chapter: How to Contemplate the Hidden Threat in the Management of Multiple Trauma Patients?

Ozgur Karcioglu and Canan Akman

1. Introduction

1.1 Case presentation

Time 05.30: after the motor-vehicle accident (MVA), a 28 year-old man has been transported to the emergency department (ED) by a taxi. The patient had been driving the vehicle himself, his seat belt was not fastened, and he smelt alcohol. He was on the ground next to the vehicle that had tumbled off the road at the time of the accident.

Time 05.52: the patient is taken to the ED. Conscious, trying to cooperate, agitated.

BP: 100/70 mmHg, pulse: 128 bpm, respiratory rate (RR): 30 bpm, arterial O_2 saturation (SaO_2, pulse oximetry): 96%.

Head – neck: there is skin abrasion in the right maxillary region. There is no cervical tenderness.

Resp: breath sounds are equal. No rales, no rhonchus. Crepitus and tenderness are detected on the right at the 10th rib level.

CVS: rhythmic, tachycardic.

Abdomen: cannot be reliably evaluated due to the patient's agitation. Voluntary guarding and tenderness in the right upper quadrant are noted. Bedside abdominal ultrasonography was difficult to interpret because of overlying bowel gas and obesity.

Extremity: open, comminuted fracture 20 cm proximal to the ankle on the right tibia and fibula. There is no pulse in the dorsalis pedis. There is external bleeding from the wound.

At 06.00: a vascular access is opened to the patient from the left antecubital region with an 18 G, and 500 mL of normal saline is infused.

Tetanus vaccine 0.5 mL IM and antibiotic prophylaxis are administered.

Complete blood count, blood group, and blood alcohol level are ordered, and blood transfusion is prepared. His chest radiography and right tibia and fibula radiographies are ordered.

The right leg is irrigated with normal saline, bandaged, and splinted, and the patient was sent to radiology suit. His tachycardia is thought to be due to pain and agitation.

07.00: the patient returns from radiology. PA chest radiograph shows a right 10th rib fracture and a communited, displaced fracture in the right tibia and fibula.

IntechOpen

BP: 90/50 mmHg, and heart rate: 130 bpm. Hemoglobin (Hb): 13.2 g/dL, and hematocrit (Htc): 38.0%. Orthopedic consultation is requested. The patient is evaluated, and hospitalization is planned for the operation. Vascular surgeon is being consulted, and angiography is planned.

Time 07.30: BP 80/40 mmHg, and heart rate: 125 bpm.

The patient's general condition deteriorates. He looks pale, sweaty, and cold. He can barely cooperate. Fluid administration is continued. Hb: 6.2 g/dL; Htc 20.1%.

Considering that the patient had blood loss from an open fracture, three units of blood were administered. Transfusion is performed. Hb is 8.5 g, and Htc is 24.5%.

While the patient is waiting for angiography, he develops hypotension and bradycardia.

Time 09.00: respiratory and cardiac arrest are observed in the patient. Resuscitation (CPR) is commenced. The patient is unresponsive. In the postmortem evaluation, it was determined that the cause of death was intra-abdominal hemorrhage due to liver laceration.

2. Approach to multiple trauma

Trauma has long been the most common cause of death and disability in the productive age group, childhood, and young adults (1–40 years) in the world, including developed countries [1]. It is an enormous social problem that disables large masses and has a significant share in healthcare costs. For the physician, it refers to a wide range of patient groups, from life-threatening and disabling injuries to pathologies that can be corrected with minor interventions.

In the evaluation of all kinds of trauma cases, a standard approach system has been introduced and has been widely accepted all over the world, regardless of the external appearance of the patient. This approach is known as Advanced Trauma Life Support (ATLS), in which the patient's care is characterized by two main parts: primary and secondary care.

In a patient with major blunt injury, the first hour is certainly the most decisive period for massive bleeding and shock [2]. Those inappreciable minutes can be used to identify the victim's clinical condition and institute specific treatments. Trauma victims with certain criteria should be transferred to developed institutions also called as trauma centers in some countries: penetrating injuries to head, neck, torso, and extremities proximal to elbow and knee, flail chest, two or more proximal long bone fractures, crushed, degloved, or mangled extremity, amputation proximal to wrist and ankle, pelvic fractures, open or depressed skull fracture, and paralysis [3].

In this approach to trauma, the team leader is a person experienced in resuscitation and is responsible for the clinical monitoring of the patient and intervention orders. In a trauma case, the emergency physician should try to rule out the patient by assuming the worst possible injury. Most of the time, treatment interventions have to be initiated in the ED before a definitive diagnosis is established. For example, in a trauma case where tension pneumothorax is suspected, needle thoracostomy is performed without waiting for a chest X-ray or blood transfusion can be initiated before the exact source of bleeding is identified.

The physician should recognize sources of life-threatening blood losses and resultant hypovolemia. Pericardial tamponade, commotio cordis, and a pneumothoraces are all difficult diagnoses to manage. These can present with hypotension associated with high readings of CVP. On the other hand, hemorrhage of thoracoabdominal viscera is most often accompanied by low blood pressure and a low levels of CVP. Emergent evaluation and treatment of thoracic trauma appears to be of vital importance, as is the utilization of the correct diagnostic strategy to evaluate the possibility of intraabdominal and retroperitoneal injury [4]. Abdominal trauma is present in approximately 25% of major trauma patients and is the leading cause of unrecognized fatal injury in children [5]. Innovative approaches such as REBOA is mostly used in most developed countries for a wide range of indications including major trauma or intraoperative bleeding.

Primary survey: it is essential to first evaluate the patient with the initials ABCDE (A: airway, B: Breathing, C: circulation, D: deficit, and E: exposure) and proceed to secondary survey if there is no pathological finding. If any pathology is detected in the primary examination, especially in the ABC (e.g., difficult breathing or tachycardia/hypotension), resuscitation procedures for the problem must be initiated before continuing the examination.

Secondary examination: a detailed physical examination should be performed (from head to toe), and pathological findings should be noted, should there be no problem in the primary examination or if an attempt has been made to solve the detected problems. If significant bleeding or neurovascular damage is detected in any extremity during the initial examination, immediate intervention should be carried out. Patients are placed on a trauma board and evaluated after a cervical collar is applied. The patient should be completely undressed before the examination, and foreign objects and contaminated clothing should be removed from the surrounding area. In a patient with suspected trauma, spinal injury should always be assumed until proven otherwise, and the patient should be immobilized. It should be shown that there is no significant injury through physical and radiological examination.

Clinicians should focus on the approach to the massively bleeding trauma patients and on the recent advances in this aspect of care. Ways to detect life-threatening, but "invisible" injuries should be instituted in this high-risk group of patients. Although the patient who has open fractures and is covered in blood and screaming and screaming due to external bleeding may seem to require urgent intervention, it should not be forgotten that the patient who has no signs of trauma and remains silent may be more urgent.

Hypocrates cited that *"thou shalt leave the cutting of the stone to the skilled craftsman"* which can be translated into the current clinical practice as "you shall leave the emergency treatment of multiple trauma victims to the appropriate team." Proper experience can help prevent the major pitfalls in trauma care and provide the optimal care for this high risk group.

Author details

Ozgur Karcioglu[1*] and Canan Akman[2]

1 Department of Emergency Medicine, Taksim Education and Research Hospital, University of Health Sciences, Istanbul, Turkey

2 Department of Emergency Medicine, Canakkale Onsekiz Mart University, Canakkale, Turkey

*Address all correspondence to: okarcioglu@gmail.com

References

[1] Rosen P, Barkin R. Emergency Medicine. Concepts and Clinical Practice. 4th ed. St. Louis: Mosby; 2000. pp. 352-367

[2] Tonglet ML, Greiffenstein P, Pitance F, Degesves S. Massive bleeding following severe blunt trauma: The first minutes that can change everything. Acta Chirurgica Belgica. 2016;**116**(1):11-15. DOI: 10.1080/00015458.2015.1136488

[3] Gross EA, Martel ML. Multiple Trauma. Rosen's Emergency Medicine: Concepts and Clinical Practice. 9th ed. Philadelphia, PA: Elsevier Inc.; 2018. 19103-2899. ISBN: 978-1-4557-0605-1

[4] Broos PL, Willaert WI. Notorious pitfalls in the care of multi-trauma patients. Acta Chirurgica Belgica. 2003;**103**(4):346-354. DOI: 10.1080/00015458.2003.11679442

[5] Ernst G. Pediatric Trauma. In: Tintinalli's Emergency Medicine a Comprehensive Study Guide, Editor-in-Chief Judith E. Tintinalli. 9th ed. New York: McGraw-Hill Education; 2020. ISBN: 978-1-26-001994-0

Chapter 2

Pelvic Trauma

Erdal Güngör

Abstract

Pelvic trauma (PT) occurs in 3% of skeletal injuries, presents significant challenges in trauma care. Among severe trauma patients admitted to primary care trauma centers, 10% exhibit pelvic fractures, often resulting from high-energy mechanisms. Pelvic fractures frequently result from high-energy mechanisms, are often associated with multisystem injuries, and can lead to catastrophic bleeding. There is a risk of serious morbidity and mortality in these injuries. According to trauma registries of many countries, unstable pelvic fractures are associated with mortality rates ranging from 8 to 32%. Their severity depends on associated nonpelvic injuries and/or hemorrhagic pelvic injuries. Prehospital and hospital management of severe pelvic trauma requires clear organizational and therapeutic strategies to control bleeding as quickly as possible. Mortality rates remain high, especially in patients with hemodynamic instability, due to rapid bleeding, difficulty in achieving hemostasis and related injuries. For these reasons, a multidisciplinary approach is important in the management of resuscitation, control of bleeding, and treatment of bone injuries, especially in the first hours of trauma. Multimodal treatment approach has become the gold standard in pelvic trauma. These include prehospital use of pelvic binders, appropriate imaging strategy, and appropriate use of surgical or interventional radiological control of bleeding.

Keywords: pelvic trauma, pelvic fractures, bleeding, shock, surgery, trauma, emergency management

1. Introduction

The pelvis, situated at the center between the lumbar region of the abdomen and the thighs, plays a vital role in supporting the weight of the upper body. Its structure encompasses the osseous pelvis, pelvic cavity, floor, and perineum. Besides its weight-bearing function, the pelvis also redistributes the weight to the lower extremities and provides anchorage for the muscles of the lower limbs and torso. It additionally safeguards the organs within the pelvic and abdominopelvic regions. Pelvic assessments, especially relevant in obstetrics and gynecology, are conducted through various techniques such as the diagonal and obstetric conjugates. Despite being rare, dislocations, hernias, and prolapses related to the pelvis are observed across diverse patient groups [1]. The pelvis serves multiple roles, primarily offering structural support and enabling a range of movements, including standing, walking, and running. Each segment of the pelvis contributes distinct functions, underscoring the importance of understanding each part to fully grasp the pelvis's overall roles [2, 3]. The pelvis's bony structure is akin to a ring, comprising the sacrum and the paired innominate bones – the ischium, ilium, and pubis [4]. It encloses the viscera of the gastrointestinal and genitourinary systems. The primary blood supply to the pelvis comes from the internal iliac arteries and their branches. The venous network mirrors the arterial system, forming a plexus along the posterior wall of the pelvis. Bleeding in pelvic fractures usually originates from the venous plexus or the spongy bone, although arterial hemorrhage, which is linked to life-threatening conditions, occurs in a substantial number of instances [5].

2. Mechanisms of pelvic injuries

The predominant causes of pelvic ring fractures are high-energy impacts, such as falls from significant heights, sports accidents, and various forms of road traffic incidents, including those involving pedestrians, motorcyclists, drivers, and bicyclists, as well as incidents where individuals are struck by vehicles [6, 7]. Upon arrival at emergency departments, approximately 10 to 15% of individuals with pelvic fractures are in a state of shock, and about one-third of these patients succumb to their injuries, leading to a recent reported mortality rate of 32% [8]. The primary reasons for these fatalities largely involve uncontrolled hemorrhage and the physiological depletion of the patient.

3. Injury assessment techniques

Upon admission, prompt radiological evaluations are conducted, typically involving supine X-rays for both the pelvis and chest, along with a Focused Assessment with Sonography for Trauma (FAST) abdominal ultrasound examination [9]. However, in cases where the patient's history, such as a falling on the feet, or physical examination provides strong indications of isolated pelvic trauma, such as pelvic ring deformity, a substantial hematoma altering the perineum's shape, or bleeding from the rectum or urethra, it is crucial to recognize that FAST has restricted diagnostic efficacy [10]. There's also a heightened risk of false positives for hemoperitoneum, particularly in the presence of a sizable retroperitoneal hematoma. In such scenarios, a total body spiral Computed Tomography (CT) scan offers superior diagnostic accuracy and can be performed swiftly, typically in under 2 minutes. This rapid and comprehensive imaging is essential in the urgent evaluation of pelvic and perineal trauma (PPT), concurrent with ongoing fluid resuscitation efforts. Ideally, patients should be swiftly transitioned from the CT scanning process to the angioembolization suite, typically within a timeframe of 10 to 20 minutes. Preparations for embolization can be simultaneously arranged in the angiography suite while the CT is being conducted.

4. Management principles for severe pelvic fractures

Treating severe pelvic fractures is a notably complex and critical aspect fort he care of trauma. These fractures often caused by high energy impacts and are typically accompanied by multisystem injuries, leading to potentially life-threatening hemorrhage. The morbidity and mortality associated with these injuries are significant, with reported mortality rates for unstable pelvic fractures ranging from 8 to 32% across various international trauma registries [11–16]. In-depth discussions on the resuscitation of severely injured patients are available elsewhere. Given the potential for substantial damage to the pelvic vasculature, relying on femoral venous access is often impractical due to concerns that infused fluids may not effectively reach the right atrium. Therefore, it is crucial to place two or more large-bore IntraVenous (IV) catheters (14–18 gauge) in the antecubital fossae or a large-size percutaneous introducer sheath in the subclavian vein to ensure adequate resuscitation for patients with severe pelvic injuries. In instances where peripheral IV catheterization proves unsuccessful, prompt placement of an intraosseous (IO) catheter in the proximal humerus is recommended as a temporary solution to guarantee sufficient IV access. The fluid resuscitation strategy should adhere to the principles of damage control resuscitation. For patients who remain hemodynamically unstable despite initial resuscitation, prioritizing bleeding control is crucial. Rapid identification of the bleeding source is vital, especially in situations where conducting a CT scan is unfeasible. Under such circumstances, pelvic and chest X-rays (CXR), along with Extended Focused Assessment with Sonography for Trauma (EFAST) are the only feasible imaging methods compatible with ongoing resuscitation and urgent decision-making for bleeding control, be it surgical or radiological. If CXR and EFAST exclude extra-pelvic causes of hemorrhagic shock, pelvic angiography is highly likely to reveal active arterial bleeding, necessitating a subsequent body CT scan with intravenous contrast, followed by angiography and embolization. In rare instances of uncontrollable hemorrhagic shock, angiography and embolization might be required directly following CXR and E-FAST to address potential massive non-pelvic hemorrhage. When pelvic trauma is accompanied by hemoperitoneum, determining the bleeding source becomes more complex, often depending on the stability of the pelvic fracture. Typically, the source of active bleeding is abdominal (70%) in cases of stable pelvic fractures and pelvic (56%) in cases of unstable fractures [17], though uncertainties persist in both scenarios. The extent of hemoperitoneum also plays a crucial role, as significant hemoperitoneum usually indicates major intra-abdominal bleeding that necessitates surgical intervention. Opting for angiographic embolization to control pelvic bleeding also facilitates the management of concurrent intra-abdominal bleeding sources, such as those resulting from hepatic, splenic, or renal injuries. The relevance of pelvic CXRs, in this context, hinges on the patient's hemodynamic stability and the presence of extra-pelvic (primarily thoracic and/or abdominal) bleeding sources. For hemodynamically stable patients, pelvic CXRs are less influential in patient management since normal findings rule out major pelvic injuries as the source of bleeding but do not discount the presence of pelvic fractures, which may be identified through CT scans.

In managing abdominal digestive tract injuries, standard treatment protocols are followed. For patients who have PPT, conducting a digital rectal examination is crucial; the presence of blood indicates a potential rectal injury, even if not visibly apparent. Diligent investigation for subperitoneal rectal injuries is vital, as undetected injuries can lead to a mortality rate of up to 50% when sepsis develops in patients with open pelvic fractures [18]. While monitoring for improvement in the patient's overall condition, they should be kept in intensive care, utilizing transcondylar leg traction and Ganz® clamp pelvic immobilization. The use of muscle relaxants (curarization) is essential for the effectiveness of external orthopedic procedures, ensuring the maintained reduction of the fracture and preventing the upward movement of a dislocated hemipelvis. Subsequent treatment of pelvic bony injuries involves iliosacral screw fixation for posterior fractures, occasionally in conjunction with realignment of the symphysis pubis. The ease of delayed percutaneous fracture fixation is enhanced when the pelvic ring fractures are preliminarily reduced [19].

5. Treatment approaches for pelvic injuries

The treatment for pelvic injuries encompasses a range of methods including pelvic binding, angiography with embolization, surgical stabilization, care for concurrent injuries, and the exploration of newer therapeutic approaches such as the use of resuscitative endovascular balloon occlusion of the aorta (REBOA) and the integration of operative and angiography facilities.

6. Pelvic binding

For the temporary stabilization of unstable pelvic fractures, the application of noninvasive external compression, known as pelvic binding (**Figure 1**), is advised. This method offers multiple advantages: it prevents further movement of the pelvis, decreases the pelvic volume which in turn helps in reducing bleeding, and alleviates discomfort for the patient [20]. Quick stabilization is possible through the circumferential wrapping of a bedsheet around the patient's pelvis, specifically positioned at the level of the greater trochanter. It's crucial to ensure the wrap is placed accurately

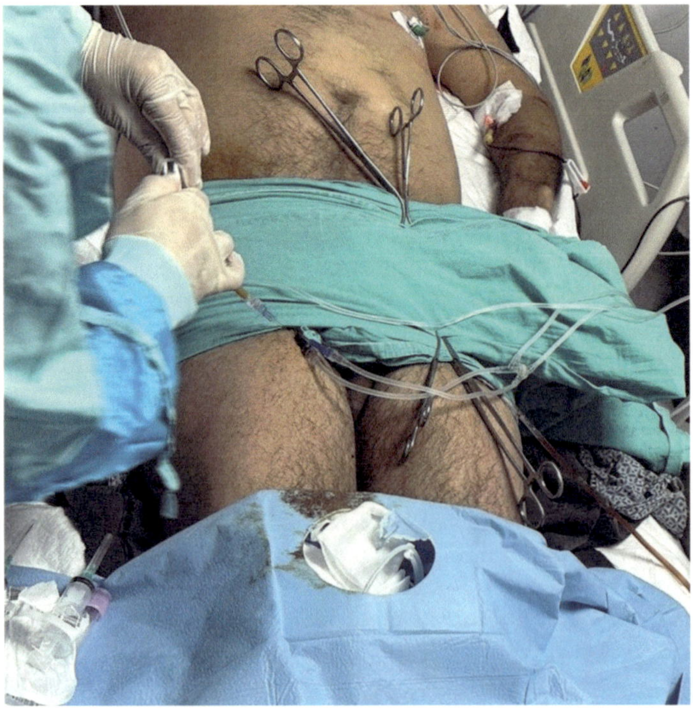

Figure 1.
Pelvic binding.

for maximum effectiveness. While there are various commercially available devices designed for pelvic binding, there is not conclusive evidence to suggest that these are superior to the use of a simple bedsheet. Some commercial devices might offer benefits in terms of ease of application and consistency [21], but they may also restrict access to the groin area which is necessary for procedures like angiography or REBOA placement. In contrast, a bedsheet can be modified to provide necessary access while still maintaining the effectiveness of the wrap. Using Kelly clamps to secure the bedsheet can help reduce the risk of skin necrosis, a common issue with knots, but it's important to note that these clamps might create artifacts in CT scans. This issue can be circumvented by opting for commercially available zip ties as an alternative for securing the wrap.

7. Extraperitoneal pelvic packing (EPP)

First introduced in literature in 1994 [22], EPP has gained increasing clinical application since the year 2000 [23–28]. EPP is recognized for its effectiveness in stabilizing patients who continue to be unstable despite traditional management methods, including skeletal fixation and arteriography. However, there is a lack of consensus regarding its role, as evidenced by differing American and European guidelines. In the United States, EPP is regarded as an effective method for hemorrhage control, but primarily as a secondary strategy following embolization, with a Grade III evidence level [21]. Conversely, European guidelines suggest an earlier use of EPP in patients who continue to bleed despite successful pelvic ring fixation or following surgical bleeding or embolization control [29]. EPP, however, is an invasive procedure, and there have been reports of surgical site infections associated with its use [26, 30], particularly when performed in trauma bay settings. Additionally, there is an increased risk of developing abdominal compartment syndrome(ACS) [24, 31] and the potential need for subsequent re-operation and removal of the packing within 24 to 48 hours.

8. Angiography and embolization

The majority of bleeding associated with pelvic fractures originates from veins; however, arterial hemorrhage, when it occurs, often gives rise to being hemodynamic instable and an increased risk of blood loss. Transcatheter Arterial Embolization (TAE) is recognized as the most effective treatment for managing pelvic fractures accompanied by arterial bleeding. Newest systematic reviews of TAE in pelvic fractures show an effectivity rate ranging from 81 to 100% in controlling arterial hemorrhage, resulting in a significant reduction in the need for blood transfusions and a decrease in mortality rates associated with pelvic bleeding [32]. Indications for TAE are ongoing hemodynamic instability, post-resuscitation and pelvic binding, the presence of a contrast enhancement on CT scans, a visible large pelvic hematoma on CT, and advanced patient age [21]. Timely execution of TAE is crucial, as delays have been associated with increased mortality risks [33, 34], presenting a critical challenge even in well-equipped trauma centers [35]. There is considerable interest in establishing the optimal sequence of interventions for controlling hemorrhage in hemodynamically unstable patients with pelvic fractures.

9. Resuscitative endovascular balloon occlusion of the aorta (REBOA)

REBOA is recognized as an innovative and effective method for controlling bleeding in patients experiencing hemorrhagic shock. Specifically, the deployment of the balloon in Zone 3 has been suggested as a viable option for managing pelvic hemorrhage [36, 37]. Studies have indicated that the use of REBOA in Zone 3, in contrast to Zone 1, significantly enhances survival rates by effectively controlling pelvic arterial blood flow [38]. Despite its potential, REBOA is not widely available, and some research has pointed to its association with serious complications, including ischemia-reperfusion syndrome, acute kidney injury, limb amputation, and an increase in mortality rates [39].

10. Operative stabilization: external pelvic fixation in hemodynamically unstable pelvic injuries

The biomechanics of pelvic ring injuries and the specific nature of the trauma largely dictate the necessity for external fixation [40, 41]. For patients with hemodynamically unstable pelvic ring injury, temporary stabilization is essential to prevent additional hemorrhage and to facilitate hemorrhage control methods such as angiography and pelvic packing [40, 42–45]. The fundamental objectives of immediate external pelvic fixation encompass diminishing intrapelvic volume in injuries resembling an "open book" configuration to mitigate the space for retroperitoneal bleeding and offering a steadfast counterpressure against lap sponges employed in pelvic packing. Notably, pelvic packing is ineffective without sufficient counterpressure from the posterior pelvic structures, necessitating external fixation in cases of unstable pelvic ring disruptions [41, 46, 47]. Determining the appropriate type of external fixation, often termed "damage control" fixation, for unstable pelvic ring injuries is a complex decision-making process [40]. The indication of pelvic external fixation are guided by the Young & Burgess fracture classification system and defined the technique [40, 48]. Anterior posterior compression and lateral compression injuries are typically addressed with anterior stabilization frames, employing either iliac crest or supra-acetabular Schanz pin application. The iliac crest approach is less technically demanding and allows for quicker application, but Schanz pins in the iliac crest have a lower resistance to pull-out, increasing the risk of fixation failure. In contrast, supra-acetabular frames, necessitating meticulous pin placement under radiographic control, offer higher pull-out resistance due to the robust supra-acetabular surgical corridor [40]. For vertically unstable pelvic ring disruptions, such as "vertical shear" (VS) injuries, a posterior C-clamp is preferred [23, 49–53]. Trauma surgeons must be cognizant of the inherent risks and technical complexities associated with the C-clamp, including a steep learning curve and the necessity for experienced application [54, 55]. Contraindications for using a pelvic C-clamp include complex sacral fractures, iliac wing fractures, and lateral compression-type injuries [40].

11. Definitive internal pelvic fixation

The optimal timing for conclusively addressing unstable pelvic ring injuries remains a topic of ongoing discussion in the medical community [56–63]. Generally, experts agree that individuals undergoing severe traumatic-hemorrhagic shock due to disruptions in the pelvic ring are typically not deemed appropriate candidates for an early definitive intervention. This is mainly because of the heightened risk of mortality linked to excessive bleeding and the potentially fatal combination of coagulopathy, acidosis, and hypothermia [64, 65]. An impactful multicenter cohort study emphasized that early fixation of pelvic fractures, especially within the initial or second day post-injury, results in significantly greater blood loss and heightened levels of interleukin (IL-6 and IL-8) in the serum, indicating an intensified systemic inflammatory response in polytrauma patients [66]. It was also noted that the early and brief period of initial pelvic stabilization contributed to a lower incidence of multiple organ failure (MOF) and reduced mortality rates [67]. However, complication rates post-injury were observed to rise when the definitive fixation of the pelvic ring was performed between the second and fourth days post-injury, compared to delaying the surgery until the sixth to eighth day [68]. The prevailing perspective endorses the strategy of initial 'damage control' external fixation for hemodynamically unstable pelvic ring injuries, followed by delayed definitive internal fixation after the fourth day, post successful resuscitation [40, 42, 69–74]. This approach, along with the application of classification systems, provides guidance in categorizing patients with unstable polytrauma and pelvic ring injuries who necessitate damage control measures, in contrast to those who are stable or borderline stable and may be suitable for an early definitive pelvic fracture intervention [59, 65]. In this context, various observational studies from the orthopedic trauma group at MetroHealth in Cleveland have shown that early fixation of pelvic fractures within 24 hours of admission in stable or borderline resuscitated patients can significantly lower the risk of complications and enhance overall outcomes [57, 59, 62, 63]. Recently, an international consensus group

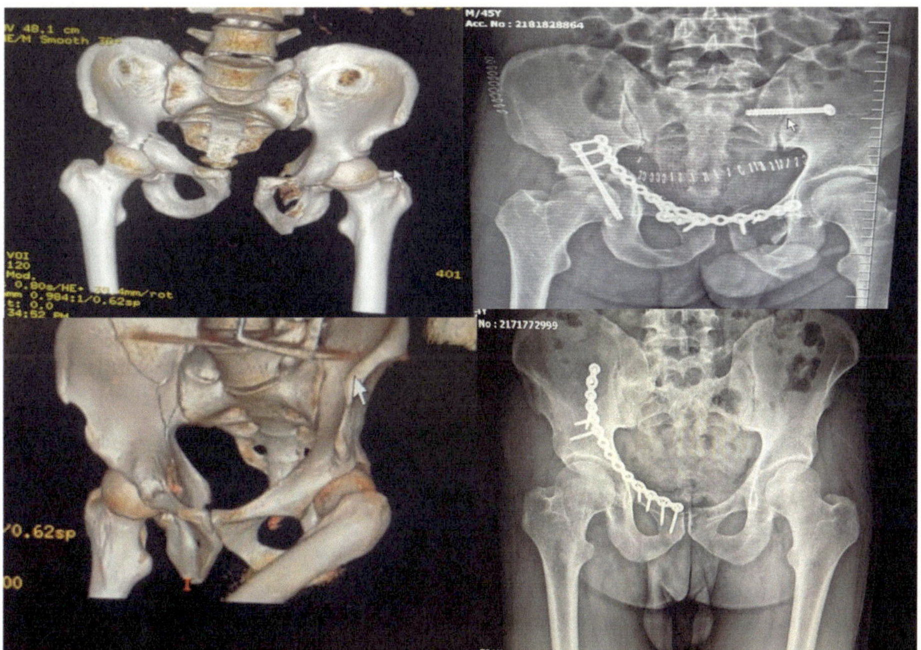

Figure 2.
Pelvic fracture with separation of pubic ramus and open reduction and fixed with plate and screws.

proposed a new definition of polytrauma, based on the severity of the injury and physiological parameter disturbances [75]. This new definition, along with recently established grading systems [59], may further refine the criteria for determining the optimal timing for definitive pelvic fracture fixation, pending additional validation studies (**Figure 2**).

12. Morbidity, mortality, and outcomes in pelvic trauma

Patients with open pelvic trauma (PT) frequently encounter complications that markedly impact functionality, giving rise to chronic consequences such as urinary and fecal incontinence, impotence, dyspareunia, residual physical disabilities, perineal and pelvic abscesses, chronic pain, and vascular complications such as embolism or thrombosis [6, 76]. It's noteworthy that the highest proportion of deaths (44.7%) occurs on the day of the trauma itself. Factors closely associated with increased mortality rates include older age, the severity of the injury as measured by the Injury Severity Score (ISS), instability of the pelvic ring, the extent and contamination of open wounds, rectal injuries, fecal diversion, the number of blood units transfused, head injury severity as per the Abbreviated Injury Scale (AIS), and the base deficit upon admission [7, 76].

A recent study has highlighted the positive impact of a multidisciplinary approach on both performance and patient outcomes [7]. Initially, a well-defined decision-making algorithm significantly reduced the time between hospital arrival and bleeding control in the theater using Pelvic Packing Procedures (PPP) [7]. Additionally, the implementation of a massive hemorrhage protocol substantially decreased the pre-transfusion administration of fluids and rationalized the use of packed red cells and fresh frozen plasma at a ratio of 2:1, commencing within the initial hours post-injury [7]. The involvement of specialized pelvic orthopedic surgeons demonstrated a significant improvement ($p = 0.004$) in the proportion of patients undergoing definitive repairs for unstable pelvic fractures, leading to enhanced patient outcomes [7]. Similar observations underscoring the importance of adhering to established guidelines were reported by Balogh et al. [77] and were subsequently reinforced by the multi-institutional trial led by Costantini et al. [8].

13. Conclusion

This chapter has highlighted key advancements in managing pelvic trauma, focusing on combatting profuse bleeding and shock, and detailing both emergency and definitive treatment strategies. Our findings emphasize the importance of immediate interventions, such as the use of pelvic binders and tranexamic acid, which have proven critical in reducing the mortality rates associated with these injuries. The study further demonstrates the effectiveness of an integrated approach combining surgical and interventional radiology techniques for rapid hemorrhage control, significantly enhancing patient stabilization.

Moreover, we have outlined improvements in definitive treatment approaches, advocating for a patient-specific strategy that optimizes mechanical stability and physiological recovery. The incorporation of a multidisciplinary framework underscores the necessity of cross-specialty collaboration for effective pelvic trauma management.

In summary, this research contributes significantly to the existing body of knowledge on pelvic trauma care, offering innovative strategies for emergency intervention and definitive treatment that promise to improve patient outcomes in trauma care settings.

Author details

Erdal Güngör
Departman of Orthopaedic and Traumatoloji, Medipol University Esenler Hospital, İstanbul, Turkey

*Address all correspondence to: egungor_49@hotmail.com

References

[1] DeSilva JM, Rosenberg KR. Anatomy, development, and function of the human pelvis. The Anatomical Record (Hoboken). 2017;**300**(4):628-632

[2] Aldabe D, Hammer N, Flack NAMS, Woodley SJ. A systematic review of the morphology and function of the sacrotuberous ligament. Clinical Anatomy. 2019;**32**(3):396-407

[3] Matsutani H, Nakai G, Yamada T, Yamamoto K, Ohmichi M, Narumi Y. Diversity of imaging features of ovarian sclerosing stromal tumors on MRI and PET-CT: A case report and literature review. Journal of Ovarian Research. 2018;**11**(1):101

[4] Marx J, Walls R, Hockberger R, Biros M, et al, editors. Rosen's Emergency Medicine - Concepts and Clinical Practice. Vol. 2014. Philadelphia, PA: Elsevier/Saunders; 2014. pp. 656-671

[5] Cook RE, Keating JF, Gillespie I. The role of angiography in the management of haemorrhage from major fractures of the pelvis. Journal of Bone and Joint Surgery. British Volume (London). 2002;**84**(2):178-182

[6] Arvieux C, Thony F, Broux C, et al. Current management of severe pelvic and perineal trauma. Journal of Visceral Surgery. 2012;**149**:e227-e238

[7] Perkins ZB, Maytham GD, Koers L, Bates P, Brohi K, Tai NR. Impact on outcome of a targeted performance improvement programme in haemodynamically unstable patients with a pelvic fracture. The Bone & Joint Journal. 2014;**96-B**:1090-1097

[8] Costantini TW, Coimbra R, Holcomb JB, et al. Current management of hemorrhage from severe pelvic fractures: Results of an American Association for the Surgery of Trauma multi-institutional trial. Journal of Trauma and Acute Care Surgery. 2016;**80**:717-723. discussion 23-25

[9] Arvieux C, Cardin N, Létoublon C. La laparotomie écourtée pour le traitement des traumatismes abdominaux sévères. In: Annales de Chirurgie. Vol. 131, No. 5. Elsevier Masson; May 2006. pp. 342-346

[10] Ballard RB, Rozycki GS, Newman PG, et al. An algorithm to reduce the incidence of false-negative FAST examinations in patients at high risk for occult injury. Focused assessment for the sonographic examination of the trauma patient. Journal of the American College of Surgeons. 1999;**189**:145-150 [discussion 141-150]

[11] Giannoudis PV, Grotz MRW, Tzioupis C, et al. Prevalence of pelvic fractures, associated injuries, and mortality: The United Kingdom perspective. The Journal of Trauma. 2007;**63**(4):875-883

[12] Hauschild O, Strohm PC, Culemann U, et al. Mortality in patients with pelvic fractures: Results from the German pelvic injury register. The Journal of Trauma. 2008;**64**(2):449-455

[13] Yoshihara H, Yoneoka D. Demographic epidemiology of unstable pelvic fracture in the United States from 2000 to 2009: Trends and in-hospital mortality. Journal of Trauma and Acute Care Surgery. 2014;**76**(2):380-385

[14] Vaidya R, Scott AN, Tonnos F, et al. Patients with pelvic fractures from blunt trauma. What is the cause of mortality and when? American Journal of Surgery. 2016;**211**(3):495-500

[15] Costantini TW, Coimbra R, Holcomb JB, et al. Current management of hemorrhage from severe pelvic fractures. Journal of Trauma and Acute Care Surgery. 2016;**80**(5):717-725

[16] Inaba K, Sharkey PW, Stephen DJG, et al. The increasing incidence of severe pelvic injury in motor vehicle collisions. Injury. 2004;**35**(8):759-765

[17] Eastridge BJ, Starr A, Minei JP, O'Keefe GE, Scalea TM. The importance of fracture pattern in guiding therapeutic decision-making in patients with hemorrhagic shock and pelvic ring disruptions. The Journal of Trauma. 2002;**53**:446-450

[18] Dente CJ, Feliciano DV, Rozycki GS, et al. The outcome of open pelvic fractures in the modern era. American Journal of Surgery. 2005;**190**:830-835

[19] Nordin J, Tonetti J. Les fractures et disjonctions de l'anneau pelvien de l'adulte. Paris: Monographie de la Sofcot; 2006. pp. 31-34

[20] Bakhshayesh P, Boutefnouchet T, Tötterman A. Effectiveness of non invasive external pelvic compression: A systematic review of the literature. Scandinavian Journal of Trauma, Resuscitation and Emergency Medicine. 2016;**24**:73

[21] Cullinane DC, Schiller HJ, Zielinski MD, et al. Eastern Association for the Surgery of trauma practice management guidelines for hemorrhage in pelvic fracture– Update and systematic review. The Journal of Trauma. 2011;**71**(6):1850-1868

[22] Pohlemann T, Bosch U, Gänsslen A, Tscherne H. The Hanover experience in management of pelvic fractures. Clinical Orthopaedics. 1994;**305**:69-80

[23] Ertel W, Eid K, Keel MTO. Therapeutical strategies and outcome of polytraumatized patients with pelvic injuries. European Journal of Trauma. 2000;**26**:278-286

[24] Ertel W, Keel M, Eid K, Platz A, Trentz O. Control of severe hemorrhage using C-clamp and pelvic packing in multiply injured patients with pelvic ring disruption. Journal of Orthopaedic Trauma. 2001;**15**(7):468-474

[25] Smith WR, Moore EE, Osborn P, et al. Retroperitoneal packing as a resuscitation technique for hemodynamically unstable patients with pelvic fractures: Report of two representative cases and a description of technique. The Journal of Trauma. 2005;**59**(6):1510-1514

[26] Cothren CC, Osborn PM, Moore EE, Morgan SJ, Johnson JL, Smith WR. Preperitonal pelvic packing for hemodynamically unstable pelvic fractures: A paradigm shift. The Journal of Trauma. 2007;**62**(4):834-839 [discussion 839-842]

[27] Pohlemann T, Gansslen A, Hufner T, Tscherne H. EXtraperitoneal packing at laparotomy. In: Abstract OTA-AAST Annual Meeting. 2000

[28] Giannoudis PV, Pape HC. Damage control orthopaedics in unstable pelvic ring injuries. Injury. 2004;**35**(7):671-677

[29] Rossaint R, Bouillon B, Cerny V, et al. Management of bleeding following major trauma: An updated European guideline. Critical Care. 2010;**14**(2):R52

[30] Tötterman A, Madsen JE, Skaga NO, Røise O. Extraperitoneal pelvic packing: A salvage procedure to control massive traumatic pelvic hemorrhage. The Journal of Trauma. 2007;**62**(4):843-852

[31] Ertel W, Oberholzer A, Platz A, Stocker R, Trentz O. Incidence and

clinical pattern of the abdominal compartment syndrome after "damage control" laparotomy in 311 patients with severe abdominal and/or pelvic trauma. Critical Care Medicine. 2000;**28**(6):1747-1753

[32] Papakostidis C, Kanakaris N, Dimitriou R, et al. The role of arterial embolization in controlling pelvic fracture haemorrhage: A systematic review of the literature. European Journal of Radiology. 2012;**81**(5):897-904

[33] Schwartz DA, Medina M, Cotton BA, et al. Are we delivering two standards of care for pelvic trauma? Availability of angioembolization after hours and on weekends increases time to therapeutic intervention. Journal of Trauma and Acute Care Surgery. 2014;**76**(1):134-139

[34] Tanizaki S, Maeda S, Matano H, et al. Time to pelvic embolization for hemodynamically unstable pelvic fractures may affect the survival for delays up to 60 min. Injury. 2014;**45**(4):738-741

[35] Tesoriero R, Bruns B, Narayan M, et al. Angiographic embolization for hemorrhage following pelvic fracture: Is it "time" for a paradigm shift? Journal of Trauma and Acute Care Surgery. 2017;**82**(1):18-26

[36] Brenner M, Teeter W, Hoehn M, Pasley J, Hu P, Yang S, et al. Use of resuscitative endovascular balloon occlusion of the aorta for proximal aortic control in patients with severe hemorrhage and arrest. JAMA Surgery. 2018;**153**:130-135

[37] Morrison JJ, Percival TJ, Markov NP, Villamaria C, Scott DJ, Saches KA, et al. Aortic balloon occlusion is effective in controlling pelvic hemorrhage. The Journal of Surgical Research. 2012;**177**:341-347

[38] Do WS, Forte DM, Sheldon RR, Weiss JB, Barron MR, Sokol KK, et al. Preperitoneal balloon tamponade and resuscitative endovascular balloon occlusion of the aorta: Alternatives to open packing for pelvic-associated hemorrhage. Journal of Trauma and Acute Care Surgery. 2019;**87**:18-26

[39] DuBose JJ, Scalea TM, Brenner M, Skiada D, Inaba K, Cannon J, et al. The AAST prospective aortic occlusion for resuscitation in trauma and acute care surgery (AORTA) registry: Data on contemporary utilization and outcomes of aortic occlusion and resuscitative balloon occlusion of the aorta (REBOA). Journal of Trauma and Acute Care Surgery. 2016;**81**:409-419

[40] Stahel PF, Mauffrey C, Smith WR, et al. External fixation for acute pelvic ring injuries: Decision making and technical options. Journal of Trauma and Acute Care Surgery. 2013;**75**:882-887

[41] Rommens PM, Hofmann A, Hessmann MH. Management of Acute Hemorrhage in pelvic trauma: An overview. European Journal of Trauma and Emergency Surgery. 2010;**36**:91-99

[42] Marzi I, Lustenberger T. Management of Bleeding Pelvic Fractures. Scandinavian Journal of Surgery. 2014;**103**:104-111

[43] Abrassart S, Stern R, Peter R. Unstable pelvic ring injury with hemodynamic instability: What seems the best procedure choice and sequence in the initial management? Orthopaedics & Traumatology, Surgery & Research. 2013;**99**:175-182

[44] Esmer E, Esmer E, Derst P, Schulz M, Siekmann H, Delank KS, et al. Influence of external pelvic stabilization on hemodynamically

unstable pelvic fractures. Der Unfallchirurg. 2017;**120**:312-319

[45] Poenaru DV, Popescu M, Anglitoiu B, Popa I, Andrei D, Birsasteanu F. Emergency pelvic stabilization in patients with pelvic posttraumatic instability. International Orthopaedics. 2015;**39**:961-965

[46] Burlew CC, Moore EE, Smith WR, et al. Preperitoneal pelvic packing/external fixation with secondary angioembolization: Optimal care for life-threatening hemorrhage from unstable pelvic fractures. Journal of the American College of Surgeons. 2011;**212**:628-635. discussion 35-37

[47] Osborn PM, Smith WR, Moore EE, et al. Direct retroperitoneal pelvic packing versus pelvic angiography: A comparison of two management protocols for haemodynamically unstable pelvic fractures. Injury. 2009;**40**:54-60

[48] Burgess A. Invited commentary: Young-Burgess classification of pelvic ring fractures: Does it predict mortality, transfusion requirements, and non-orthopaedic injuries? Journal of Orthopaedic Trauma. 2010;**24**:609

[49] Lustenberger T, Fau MC, Benninger E, Fau BE, Lenzlinger PM, Lenzlinger Pm F, et al. C-clamp and pelvic packing for control of hemorrhage in patients with pelvic ring disruption. Journal of Emergencies, Trauma, and Shock. 2011;**4**:477-482

[50] Heini PF, Witt J, Ganz R. The pelvic C-clamp for the emergency treatment of unstable pelvic ring injuries. A report on clinical experience of 30 cases. Injury. 1996;**27**(Suppl. 1):S-A38-S-A45

[51] Pohlemann T, Culemann U, Tosounidis G, Kristen A. Application of the pelvic C-clamp. Der Unfallchirurg. 2004;**107**:1185-1191

[52] Tiemann AH, Schmidt C, Gonschorek O, Josten C. Use of the "c-clamp" in the emergency treatment of unstable pelvic fractures. Zentralblatt für Chirurgie. 2004;**129**:245-251

[53] Witschger P, Heini P, Ganz R. Pelvic clamps for controlling shock in posterior pelvic ring injuries. Application, biomechanical aspects and initial clinical results. Der Orthopäde. 1992;**21**:393-399

[54] Koller H, Balogh ZJ. Single training session for first time pelvic C-clamp users: Correct pin placement and frame assembly. Injury. 2012;**43**:436-439

[55] Koller H, Keil P, Seibert F. Individual and team training with first time users of the pelvic C-clamp: Do they remember or will we need refresher trainings? Archives of Orthopaedic and Trauma Surgery. 2013;**133**:343-349

[56] Balbachevsky D, Belloti JC, Doca DG, et al. Treatment of pelvic fractures—A national survey. Injury. 2014;**45**(Suppl. 5):S46-S51

[57] Childs BR, Nahm NJ, Moore TA, Vallier HA. Multiple procedures in the initial surgical setting: When do the benefits outweigh the risks in patients with multiple system trauma? Journal of Orthopaedic Trauma. 2016;**30**:420-425

[58] Enninghorst N, Toth L, King KL, McDougall D, Mackenzie S, Balogh ZJ. Acute definitive internal fixation of pelvic ring fractures in polytrauma patients: A feasible option. The Journal of Trauma. 2010;**68**:935-941

[59] Nahm NJ, Moore TA, Vallier HA. Use of two grading systems in determining risks associated with timing of fracture fixation. Journal of Trauma and Acute Care Surgery. 2014;**77**:268-279

[60] Pape HC, Tornetta P 3rd, Tarkin I, Tzioupis C, Sabeson V, Olson SA. Timing of fracture fixation in multitrauma patients: The role of early total care and damage control surgery. The Journal of the American Academy of Orthopaedic Surgeons. 2009;**17**:541-549

[61] Schreiber VM, Tarkin IS, Hildebrand F, et al. The timing of definitive fixation for major fractures in polytrauma–a matched-pair comparison between a US and European level I centres: Analysis of current fracture management practice in polytrauma. Injury. 2011;**42**:650-654

[62] Vallier HA, Cureton BA, Ekstein C, Oldenburg FP, Wilber JH. Early definitive stabilization of unstable pelvis and acetabulum fractures reduces morbidity. The Journal of Trauma. 2010;**69**:677-684

[63] Vallier HA, Moore TA, Como JJ, et al. Complications are reduced with a protocol to standardize timing of fixation based on response to resuscitation. Journal of Orthopaedic Surgery and Research. 2015;**10**:155

[64] Stahel PF, Moore EE, Schreier SL, Flierl MA, Kashuk JL. Transfusion strategies in postinjury coagulopathy. Current Opinion in Anaesthesiology. 2009;**22**:289-298

[65] Pape HC, Giannoudis PV, Krettek C, Trentz O. Timing of fixation of major fractures in blunt polytrauma: Role of conventional indicators in clinical decision making. Journal of Orthopaedic Trauma. 2005;**19**:551-562

[66] Pape HC, Griensven MV, Hildebrand FF, et al. Systemic inflammatory response after extremity or truncal fracture operations. The Journal of Trauma. 2008;**65**:1379-1384

[67] Probst C, Probst T, Gaensslen A, Krettek C, Pape HC. Timing and duration of the initial pelvic stabilization after multiple trauma in patients from the German trauma registry: Is there an influence on outcome? The Journal of Trauma. 2007;**62**:370-377. discussion 6-7

[68] Pape H, Stalp M, Griensven M, Weinberg A, Dahlweit M, Tscherne H. Optimal timing for secondary surgery in polytrauma patients: An evaluation of 4314 serious-injury cases. Der Chirurg. 1999;**70**:1287-1293

[69] Spanjersberg WR, Knops SP, Schep NW, van Lieshout EM, Patka P, Schipper IB. Effectiveness and complications of pelvic circumferential compression devices in patients with unstable pelvic fractures: A systematic review of literature. Injury. 2009;**40**:1031-1035

[70] Halawi MJ. Pelvic ring injuries: Emergency assessment and management. Journal of Clinical Orthopaedics and Trauma. 2015;**6**:252-258

[71] Chu CH, Tennakoon L, Maggio PM, Weiser TG, Spain DA, Staudenmayer KL. Trends in the management of pelvic fractures, 2008-2010. The Journal of Surgical Research. 2016;**202**:335-340

[72] D'Alleyrand JC, O'Toole RV. The evolution of damage control orthopedics: Current evidence and practical applications of early appropriate care. The Orthopedic Clinics of North America. 2013;**44**:499-507

[73] Katsoulis E, Giannoudis PV. Impact of timing of pelvic fixation on functional outcome. Injury. 2006;**37**:1133-1142

[74] Pape HC, Giannoudis P, Krettek C. The timing of fracture treatment in polytrauma patients: Relevance of

damage control orthopedic surgery. American Journal of Surgery. 2002;**183**:622-629

[75] Pape HC, Lefering R, Butcher N, et al. The definition of polytrauma revisited: An international consensus process and proposal of the new 'Berlin definition'. Journal of Trauma and Acute Care Surgery. 2014;**77**:780-786

[76] Grotz MR, Allami MK, Harwood P, Pape HC, Krettek C, Giannoudis PV. Open pelvic fractures: Epidemiology, current concepts of management and outcome. Injury. 2005;**36**:1-13

[77] Balogh Z, Caldwell E, Heetveld M, et al. Institutional practice guidelines on management of pelvic fracture-related hemodynamic instability: Do they make a difference? The Journal of Trauma. 2005;**58**:778-782

Chapter 3

Eco-Guided Ankle Block: Analgesia and Anesthetic Technique for Foot Surgery

Alberto De La Espriella

Abstract

Regional anesthesia for foot surgery has become increasingly popular, there are different reasons including: most surgeries are ambulatory, great pain management during the early postoperative phase, reduced time spent in the post-anesthesia care unit, and minimizing opioid use during the perioperative period are achieved through effective ankle blockade. This procedure involves blocking the five nerves responsible for sensory supply to the area below the malleoli. It can be used both as an anesthetic technique (used together with general or neuraxial anesthesia), as well as analgesia in the context of multimodal analgesia providing adequate post-operative analgesia. All five nerves can be blocked using ultrasonography, allowing for lower latency and a smaller volume of local anesthetic.

Keywords: anesthesia, ultrasonography, nerve block, ankle, tibial nerve block, peroneal nerve block, sural nerve block, saphenous nerve block, regional anesthesia

1. Introduction

Regional anesthesia for foot surgery has become increasingly popular, there are different reasons including: most surgeries are ambulatory, great pain management during the early postoperative phase, reduced time spent in the post-anesthesia care unit, and minimizing opioid use during the perioperative period [1–3]. Foot surgery is a common procedure, and the patient population undergoing it represents a cross-section of society.

Foot surgery presents a challenge due to the intense postoperative pain, which is often difficult to manage despite employing balanced multimodal analgesia involving medications like paracetamol, non-steroidal-anti-inflammatory drugs (NSAIDs), and opioids [4]. The acute postoperative pain persists considerably beyond 24 hours [5]. After forefoot surgery, approximately 80% of patients endure severe pain, and about 32% experience nausea during the postoperative phase [6]. A majority of patients necessitate high doses of opioids for pain management following foot and ankle surgery [7].

The ankle block plays a pivotal role in multimodal analgesia, in many feet surgical procedures, the performance of this block is considered the first-option regional analgesic technique [8].

The recently adoption of enhanced recovery and ambulatory programs after fast-track orthopedic surgery protocols has sparked a renewed interest in ankle blocks [9].

Foot surgery typically involves regional anesthesia, commonly through a distal Sciatic Nerve block, occasionally complemented by a Saphenous Nerve block. These procedures may be conducted as single-shot injections or via catheter placement for continuous delivery of anesthesia [10]. The primary issue associated with the distal Sciatic Nerve block is its impact on motor function. This motor block leads to weakness in knee movement and foot mobility, potentially resulting in a higher risk of ankle sprains and inpatient falls. Difficulty in walking unassisted may prolong hospital stays or hinder prompt ambulation [11]. And therefore, delays postoperative mobilization, which is important in the context of ambulatory patients and when bilateral procedures are required [12]. Postoperative pain management using oral NSAIDs or opioids could potentially be harmful to organs and might have a negative impact on bone healing [13–15]. The existing perioperative pain management approaches for ankle and hindfoot surgeries may not always align with the fundamental principles of contemporary perioperative pain therapy, which involve ensuring efficient pain relief throughout the perioperative phase, facilitating early patient mobilization, and reducing adverse effects [16].

The ankle block entails blocking the five nerves responsible for sensory innervation to the area distal to the malleoli. It serves as an anesthesia method for foot surgery, provided a pneumatic tourniquet is not utilized during the procedure. Alternatively, it can be combined with general or neuraxial anesthesia to ensure sufficient analgesia in the postoperative phase [17]. If a tourniquet is required for the procedure, it is also proposed to use it at the ankle level, with good tolerance when ankle block is used as the sole anesthetic technique [18]. This approach minimally impacts motor function as it primarily targets the intrinsic muscles of the foot. Moreover, the use of long-acting local anesthetics enables extended postoperative analgesia [19].

Traditionally, the Ankle block has been conducted using landmark guidance, but there is a growing preference for ultrasound guidance [11]. These blind superficial infiltrations were very painful for the patient due to the need for high volumes of local anesthetics. In contrast, ultrasound-guided injections, unlike landmark-guided procedures relying on field infiltration, reduce discomfort associated with ankle block and enhance success rates [11].

The anatomical landmarks technique has reported high success rates (89–100%) [20, 21]; however, it has been perceived as technically challenging and unreliable. Various anatomical variations among the nerves could result in failure when employing a blind technique [22]. Additionally, it frequently encounters failure due to two primary reasons: first, a lack of comprehensive understanding regarding the fascial layers and the positioning of the five nerves relative to these fascias around the ankle; second, physicians occasionally overlook the necessity of blocking all five nerves, disregarding the fact that the sensory innervation areas of the foot partially overlap, and this overlap is not consistently predictable [23].

2. Indication (patient selection)

1. Anesthesia and pain management for surgical procedures involving the foot distal to the malleoli, particularly focusing on the forefoot, encompassing surgeries such as hallux valgus repair, forefoot arthroplasty, reconstruction, osteotomy, and amputation [24].

2. Perineural injections targeting the nerves around the foot and ankle may be proposed either for diagnostic purposes or as therapeutic interventions for individuals experiencing neuropathic pain, especially in cases involving peripheral nerve damage or entrapment [24].

3. For ankle surgeries, there is limited research on the effectiveness of local intraoperative infiltration. While some studies have demonstrated its efficacy in postoperative pain management, it does not provide intraoperative pain relief or eliminate the need for general anesthesia [25, 26]. Conversely, ankle block is a widely recognized regional anesthesia method for surgeries below the ankle [17, 27]. However, it is not suitable for procedures directly involving the ankle joint as the relevant nerve fibers exit their nerve roots 5–10 cm above the ankle joint.

The ankle block primarily involves infiltration and does not necessitate the elicitation of paresthesia; thus, patient cooperation is not mandatory. While it is most efficient for the anesthesiologist if the patient can assume both prone and supine positions, this is not essential [28].

Comparing ultrasound-guided and anatomical point techniques for ankle block, ultrasound has been shown to enhance clinical effectiveness, providing greater surgical anesthesia, reducing systemic opioid rescue requirements, and lowering total opioid doses in the postoperative period [29].

3. Contraindication

1. When surgeons need prolonged tourniquet application [24].

2. Ankle block is challenging in patients with difficult atomical landmarks, such as severe edema, multiple scars, or peripheral vascular disease [24].

3. In cases of local infection at the injection site [24].

4. Anatomy

The sensory innervation below the malleoli originates from five nerves: the tibial, superficial peroneal, deep peroneal, sural, and saphenous. These nerves are all derived from the sciatic nerve, except for the saphenous nerve (which is the terminal sensory branch of the femoral nerve) [11].

Blood vessels accompany the deep peroneal, posterior tibial, saphenous, and sural nerves, providing valuable anatomical landmarks for ultrasound-guided approaches (**Figure 1**) [30]. The sensory innervation regions corresponding to each nerve in the foot are illustrated in (**Figure 2**) [30]. While it has been suggested that the saphenous nerve may be necessary in only 3% of patients undergoing foot surgery [23], it is recommended to perform a complete block rather than a selective one, regardless of the type of surgery, due to frequent overlap in nerve territories [17].

4.1 Tibial nerve

This nerve exhibits mixed characteristics, encompassing both sensory and motor functions. It holds the distinction of being the largest nerve among the group of five

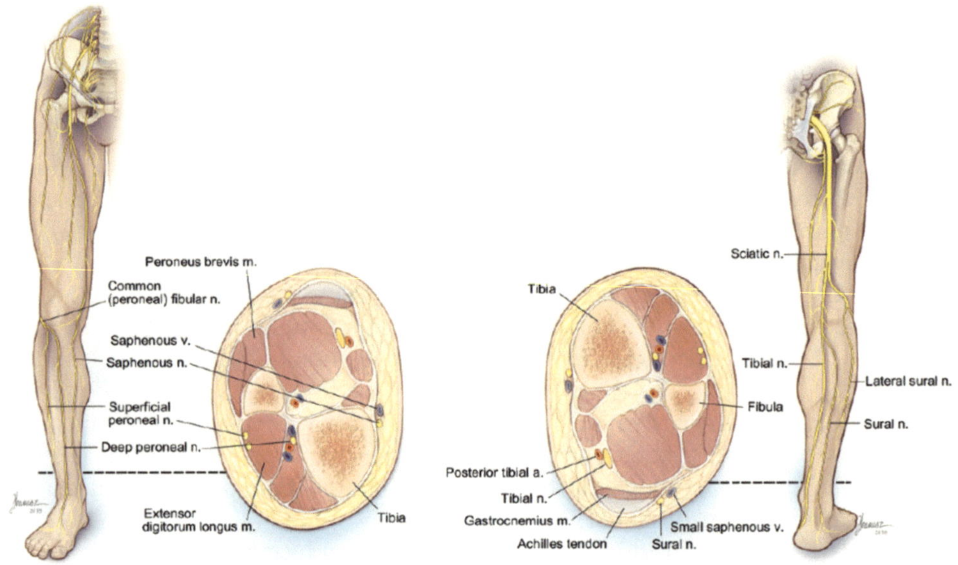

Figure 1.
Image of the anterior and posterior leg showing the course of the nerves as well as a cross section of the leg showing the location of the nerves in relationship to arteries, veins, muscles, and bones. The tibia is medial and anterior, and the fibula is lateral. Source: Ref. [28].

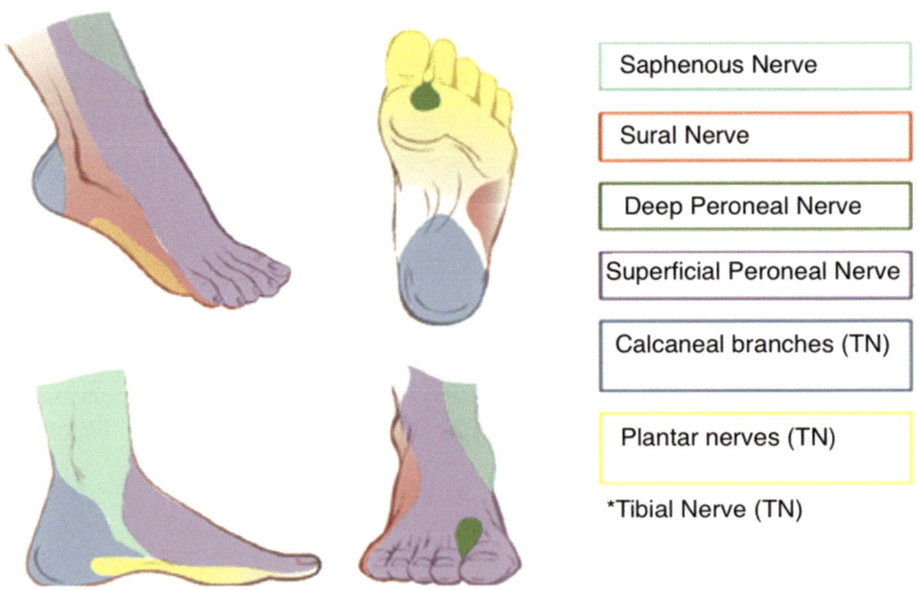

Figure 2.
Ankle block—Peripheral innervation. Source: Ref. [30].

nerves responsible for innervating the foot [31]. This nerve supplies sensation to the entire bottom surface (both bones and skin) of the foot, as well as the top surface of the first phalanx of the first, second, and half of the third toe [32]. In the ankle region, it is a direct extension of the tibial nerve beyond the point where the sciatic nerve splits in the popliteal fossa. Descending through the calf, it lies between the

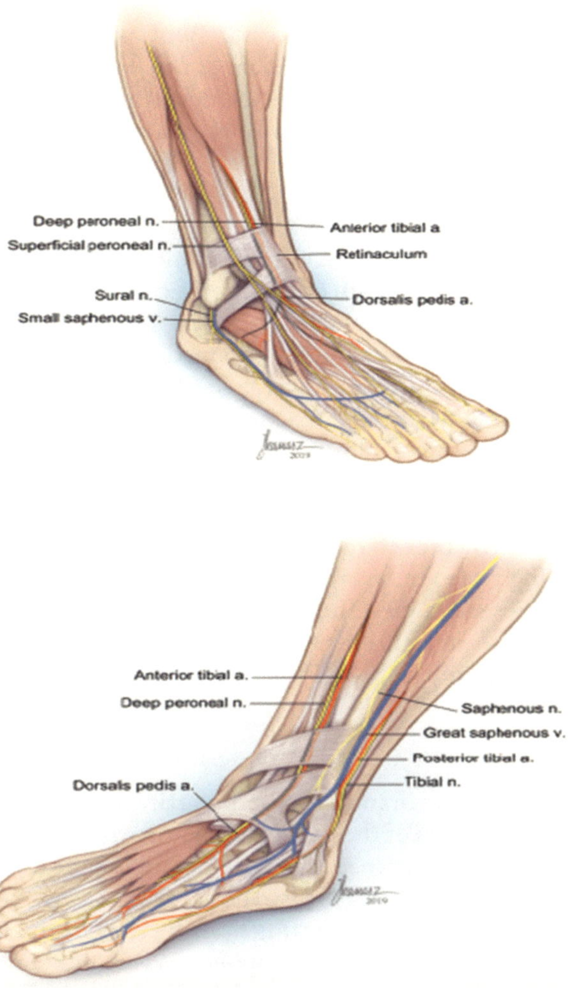

Figure 3.
Image of the lateral and medial ankle showing the course of the nerves in relationship to arteries and veins. Source: Ref. [28].

gastrocnemius/soleus muscles and the deep flexors. As it continues down the leg, it passes posterior to the medial malleolus and beneath the flexor retinaculum, typically located behind the artery. It sends branches to the medial heel (medial calcaneal branches) and eventually divides into two terminal branches: the medial and lateral plantar nerves, which innervate the sole of the foot, providing its sensory supply (**Figure 3**) [21].

4.2 Superficial peroneal (fibular) nerve

This nerve originates from the common peroneal (fibular) nerve and traverses through the peroneus longus muscle before coursing between the peroneus longus and brevis muscles. In the lower leg, it travels between the peroneus brevis and extensor digitorum longus (EDL) muscles, within the intermuscular septum that separates the anterior and lateral compartments of the leg. Its trajectory gradually shifts to a more superficial position as it progresses, ultimately piercing the crural fascia. At a subcutaneous or subfascial level, it divides into two branches: the larger medial dorsal cutaneous nerve and the smaller intermediate dorsal cutaneous nerve. These branches provide sensory innervation to the skin on the dorsal aspect of the foot and toes, covering a significant portion of the foot's dorsal surface (**Figure 3**) [24].

4.3 Deep peroneal (fibular) nerve

The deep peroneal nerve, a branch of the common peroneal nerve, originates at the fibular neck, paralleling the path of the superficial peroneal nerve. This nerve runs between the tibialis anterior muscle and the extensor hallucis longus (EHL) muscle toward the ankle, where it divides into medial and lateral branches. The medial branch continues its course alongside the dorsalis pedis artery to the first interosseous space. Passing beneath the extensor hallucis brevis tendon, it extends to the distal end of the interosseous space, where it merges with a strand of the superficial peroneal nerve (SPN) before branching into terminals for the dorsal surfaces of the first and second toes, although anatomical variations exist [33].

Conversely, the lateral branch turns outward to innervate the extensor digitorum brevis muscle, giving rise to three interosseous nerves. It supplies sensation to the area between the first and second toes, the lateral aspect of the first toe, and the medial aspect of the second toe, in addition to providing innervation to the bones on the dorsal side of the foot (**Figure 3**) [24].

4.4 Sural nerve

This nerve is formed from branches of both the tibial nerve and the common peroneal nerve at the junction of the gastrocnemius in the upper third of the calf. Specifically, the medial sural cutaneous nerve emerges in the proximal part of the popliteal fossa, descending between the two heads of the gastrocnemius muscle. It then combines with the peroneal communicating branch (lateral sural nerve) to create the sural nerve. Traveling alongside the small saphenous vein, the sural nerve passes behind the lateral malleolus within the same superficial fascial sheath. Continuing as the lateral dorsal cutaneous nerve along the lateral aspect of the foot, it sends a connecting branch to the intermediate dorsal cutaneous nerve. Ultimately, it terminates as the dorsalis digiti minimi nerve on the lateral edge of the dorsum of the small toe (**Figure 3**).

Behind the lateral malleolus, it branches into the lateral calcaneal branches, providing sensory supply to the skin in that area and at the heel. Additionally, branches for the lateral side of the ankle, the anterior capsular wall, and the tarsal sinus originate proximal to the malleolus [24].

It offers sensory innervation to the lateral aspect of the heel, the outer malleolus, and the dorsal side of the 5th and 4th toes, often extending to the 3rd toe (**Figure 3**) [34].

4.5 Saphenous nerve

The saphenous nerve is distinctive in its origin from the lumbar plexus, serving as the terminal branch of the femoral nerve. Below the knee, it runs along the tibial surface in close proximity to the great saphenous vein. The positioning of the nerve relative to the vein may vary, with the nerve situated either posteriorly or anteriorly to the vein. In the distal third of the calf, a common fascia encloses both the vein and the nerve. As it descends into the lower leg, the saphenous nerve follows a path along the medial side and anterior to the medial malleolus, emitting branches to the skin of the medial aspect of the foot. Typically, it ends in the metatarsal area without extending to the big toe. Providing sensory innervation to the medial part of the ankle and foot, it extends up to the head of the first metatarsal [32]. The extent of skin innervation may vary, with an average distance of 6.5 cm from the medial malleolus, though it may exceed 9 cm in certain cases .

There are reports of the saphenous nerve reaching deep to the periosteum of the distal tibia, the capsule of the medial malleolus in the ankle joint, and in some instances, the capsule of the talocalcaneonavicular junction in the medial area (**Figure 3**) [35].

5. Technique—Ultrasound-guided approach

5.1 Preparation for the block

Prior to the procedure, it is imperative to provide comprehensive information to the patient. Since the nerves are located superficially, a 25–50 mm 25-G needle should be sufficient [24]. The patient can be positioned supine with a footrest or pillow under the calf. During the block, the leg may need to be rotated internally or externally depending on the nerve being targeted. The proceduralist may find it efficient to maneuver around the foot while performing the block. The entire foot should be thoroughly cleaned, and the procedure must be conducted using sterile technique [28].

A high-frequency linear ultrasound probe is employed, starting at a depth of 2 cm. Long-acting local anesthetics such as 0.5–0.75% ropivacaine, 0.25–0.5% bupivacaine, or a combination of 2% lidocaine and 0.5% bupivacaine in a 1:1 ratio are utilized [24].

Regarding the volume of local anesthetic, a recommended volume of 5 ml is advised for each nerve, except for the tibial nerve, for which a volume of 5–10 ml is used due to its larger size. The literature generally advocates for a total volume ranging between 30 and 40 ml [12, 17, 23, 29]. With respect to the approach, for the five nerves a technique can be performed outside or inside the plane, recommendations varying among literature based on authors' experiences [12, 31].

This total volume aligns closely with the volume used in ankle block procedures for anatomical issues. Fredrickson et al. [36] studied 72 patients undergoing foot surgery who received ankle blocks. They were divided into two groups: one using a low volume of local anesthetic (approximately 16 ml) and the other using the conventional total volume (30 ml). The authors concluded that while a low volume resulted in a high success rate compared to the conventional volume, there might be a compromise in the duration of postoperative analgesia.

5.2 Sonoanatomy and injection technique

5.2.1 Tibial nerve

The patient is positioned supine with the hip externally rotated, allowing the medial side of the ankle to face upward. Placing the ultrasound probe in a transverse orientation between the medial malleolus and the Achilles tendon (**Figure 4**) facilitates visualization. The primary landmark for this procedure is the posterior tibial artery, often accompanied by two venae comitantes. The tibial nerve is visualized as a hyperechoic structure, typically located behind the artery and resting on the fascia of the flexor hallucis longus (FHL), although occasional anterior placement is possible. To aid in identification, the tibial nerve can be observed moving up and down

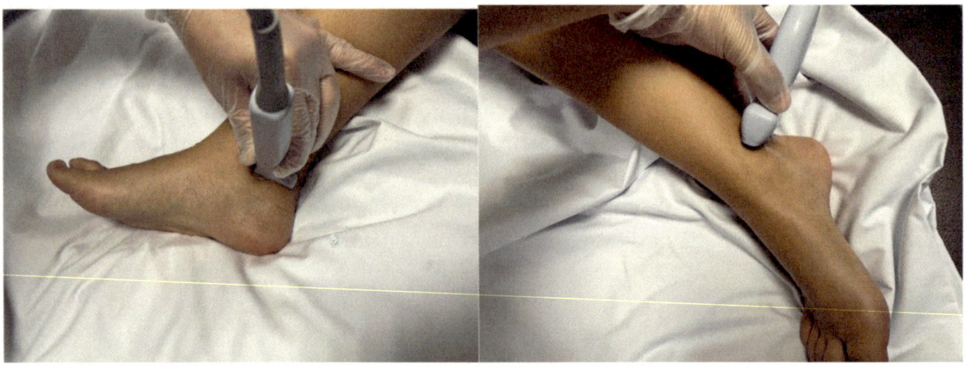

Figure 4.
Position of the patient and the transducer for tibial nerve block. Source: Authors.

by extending and flexing the big toe, as demonstrated in **Figure 5**. Performing this block proximal to the prominence of the medial malleolus is recommended to ensure sufficient blockade of the calcaneal branch [37].

Care should be taken to differentiate the flexor hallucis longus tendon, which lies deep to the tibial nerve and may be mistaken for a nerve structure due to similar sonoanatomical characteristics [30].

Both the in-plane and out-of-plane needle approaches to the nerve are viable options. The nerve is enveloped within a fascial sheath, and injecting the local anesthetic within this sheath leads to a distinctive circumferential spread of the anesthetic around the nerve. The author prefers the in-plane technique, guiding the needle into the space behind the nerve created between the flexor retinaculum and the fascia of the flexor hallucis longus. Typically, 8 to 10 ml of local anesthetic is adequate to achieve a satisfactory block.

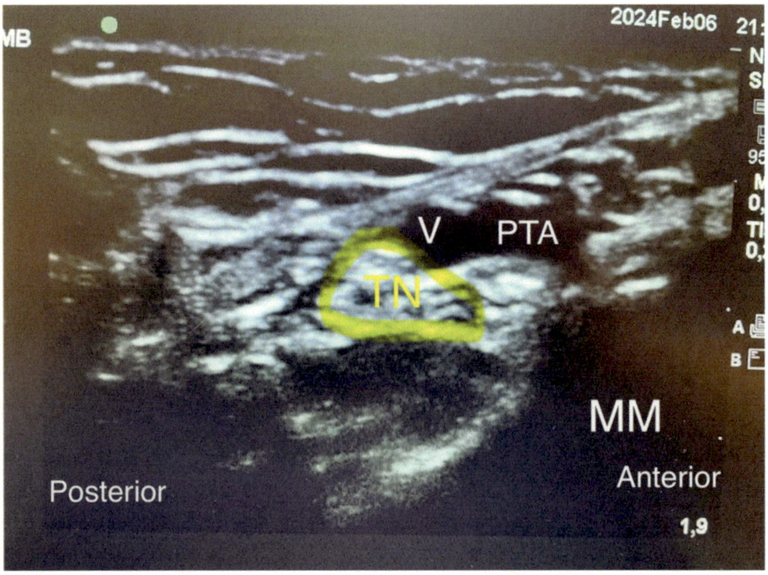

Figure 5.
Sonography of the tibial nerve at the level of medial malleolus (MM). From anterior to posterior, the structures are tibialis posterior tendon (TP), flexor digitorum, posterior tibial artery (A) and veins (V), tibial nerve (TN). Source: Authors.

In a study by Redborg et al. [38], a prospective randomized controlled trial was conducted involving 18 healthy volunteers. This study investigated the efficacy of the anatomical landmark technique versus the ultrasound-guided technique for tibial nerve block. The findings revealed a greater proportion of complete blocks at 30 minutes with ultrasound guidance (72% vs. 22%).

5.2.2 Saphenous nerve

The patient is positioned with the hip externally rotated, and the transducer is placed proximal to the medial malleolus, aligning with the position used for tibial nerve scanning (**Figure 6**) . The probe is gently positioned just above the medial malleolus in the approximate location of the greater saphenous vein. While the saphenous nerve, a small hyperechoic structure, may not always be clearly visible and does not consistently relate to the vein, the great saphenous vein serves as a reference point (**Figure** 7). In cases where the saphenous nerve is not visualized, a tourniquet can be applied around the calf to enhance venous filling (**Figure 8**).

During injection, the saphenous nerve may appear as a small hyperechoic structure superficial and posterior to the great saphenous vein. However, its visibility can vary, and in such instances, the primary landmark is the vein, and light pressure should be applied with the ultrasound probe [39]. The target area is the plane around the vein, and the needle can be inserted either in-plane or out-of-plane. Usually, a volume of 3–5 ml of local anesthetic is administered.

5.2.3 Deep peroneal (fibular) nerve

The patient is positioned supine with the leg in a neutral position. The ultrasound probe is placed transversely on the anterior surface of the ankle at the intermalleolar line, which is proximal to the ankle joint (**Figure 9**). The primary landmark for this

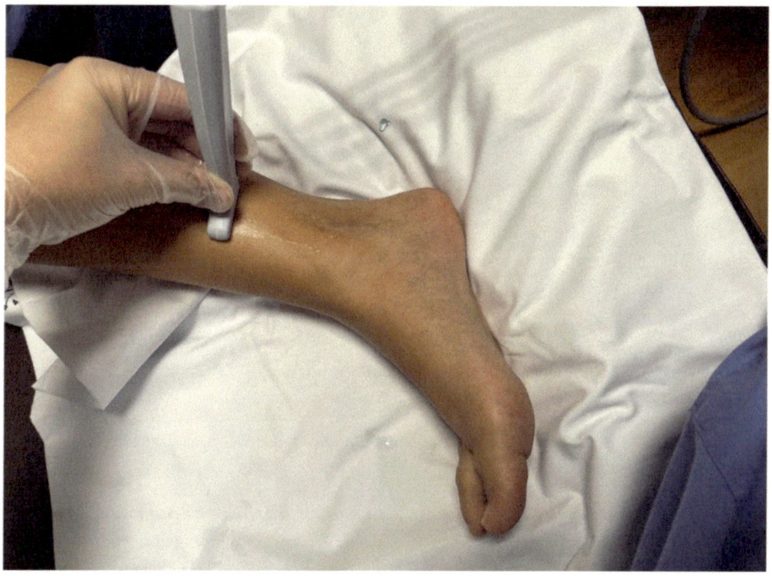

Figure 6.
Patient position and transducer for saphenous nerve block. Source: Authors.

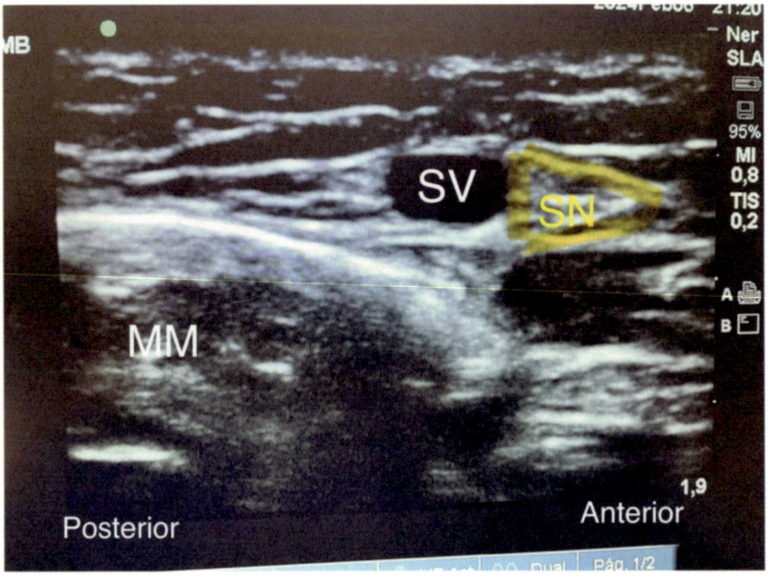

Figure 7.
Sonography of the saphenous nerve (SN) at the level of medial malleolus. It lies within the same fascia plane with the greater saphenous vein (SV). Source: Author.

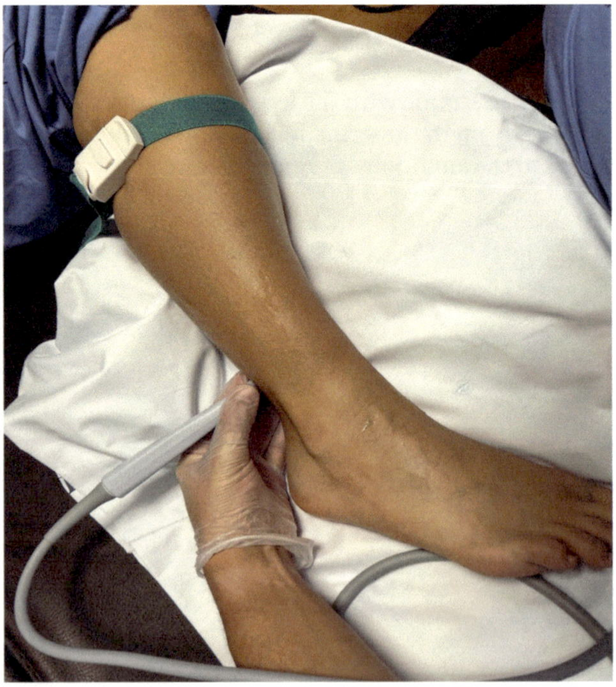

Figure 8.
A tourniquet can be placed around the calf to enhance the venous filling. Source: Author.

procedure is the anterior tibial/dorsalis pedis artery, typically located deep to the extensor hallucis longus. While the deep peroneal nerve (DPN) may sometimes appear as a small hyperechoic structure lateral to the artery in the same tissue plane, its

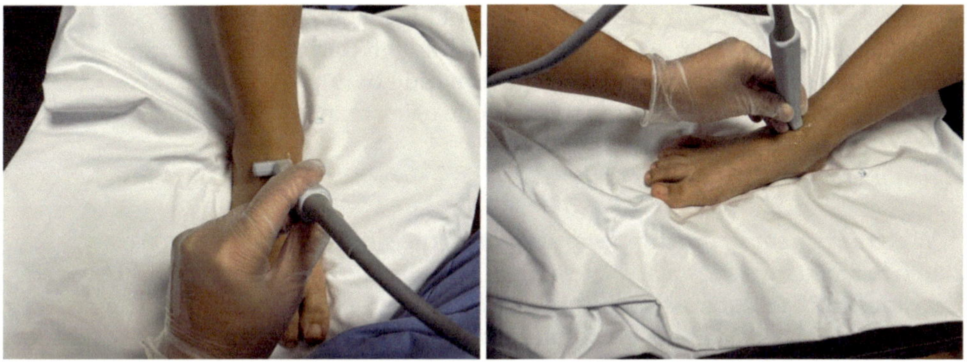

Figure 9.
Patient position and transducer for deep peroneal (fibular) nerve block. Source: Authors.

visualization is not essential for performing the block. The main purpose of visualizing the nerve is to avoid inadvertently puncturing it with the block needle (**Figure 10**), as surrounding the artery with local anesthetic ensures nerve blockade [24].

Both in-plane and out-of-plane needle approaches can be employed, with the out-of-plane approach offering a more direct needle entry for a superficial nerve. The needle tip should be directed to either side of the artery, and local anesthetic should be injected to distend the plane in which the artery lies. Care should be taken not to apply excessive pressure on the transducer, as this may occlude the artery and hinder adequate visualization. Typically, 3–5 ml of local anesthetic is adequate for achieving effective blockade.

Antonakakis et al. [40] conducted a prospective, randomized, controlled study involving 18 healthy volunteers to compare the technique for anatomical

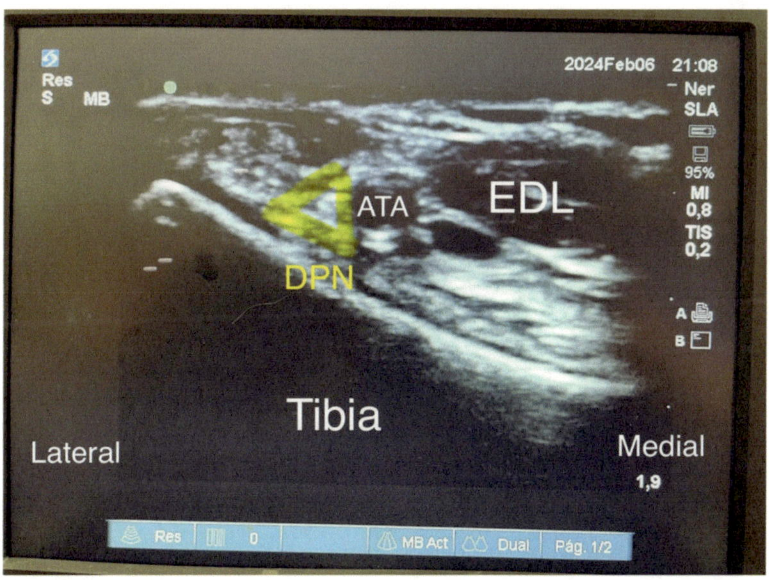

Figure 10.
Ultrasound still of the deep peroneal nerve and surrounding anatomy. Sonography of deep peroneal (fibula) nerve (DPN) at the low tibia area. The nerve is seen lateral to the anterior tibial (dorsalis pedis) artery (ATA) which is deep to the extensor digitorum longus (EDL). Source: Authors.

landmark-based blocks with the ultrasound-guided technique for deep peroneal nerve blockade. The authors concluded that although the use of ultrasound for deep peroneal nerve block reduced latency times, it did not improve the quality of the final block compared to the conventional technique using anatomical landmarks.

5.2.4 Superficial peroneal (fibular) nerve

With the patient in the supine position, the knee is flexed and the hip is internally rotated to facilitate access to the lateral aspect of the leg. Alternatively, the patient can be positioned in the lateral decubitus position, with the procedural side facing upward (**Figure 11**). The ultrasound (US) probe is placed transversely on the lateral aspect of the mid-leg, positioned above the subcutaneous part of the fibula. The fibula serves as the anatomical reference point, generating a rectangular echo. The superficial peroneal nerve is visualized as a small triangular hyperechoic structure situated within the intermuscular septum between the peroneus brevis and extensor digitorum longus muscles, just beneath the crural fascia (**Figure 12**). Its identity can be confirmed by moving the probe distally and observing the nerve emerging through the crural fascia, eventually becoming more prominent in a superficial location [41, 42].

The nerve can be blocked at the point where it lies superficial to the crural fascia, using either an in-plane or out-of-plane approach. The in-plane approach is typically preferred as it allows for easier needle entry into the narrow fascial plane. A volume of 5 ml of local anesthetic is generally sufficient to achieve a satisfactory block.

5.2.5 Sural nerve

The patient is positioned in the lateral decubitus position with the knee flexed and the hip internally rotated. The ultrasound probe is positioned transversely across

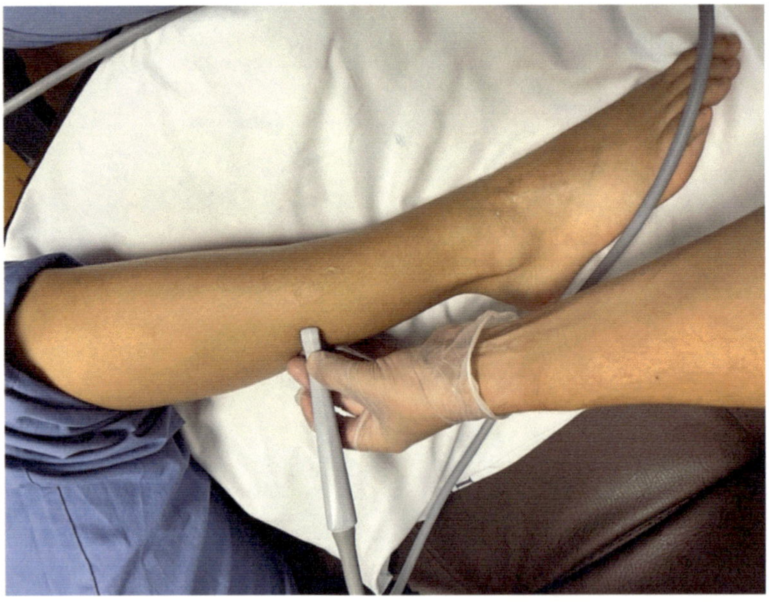

Figure 11.
Patient position and transducer for superficial peroneal (fibular) nerve block. Source: Authors.

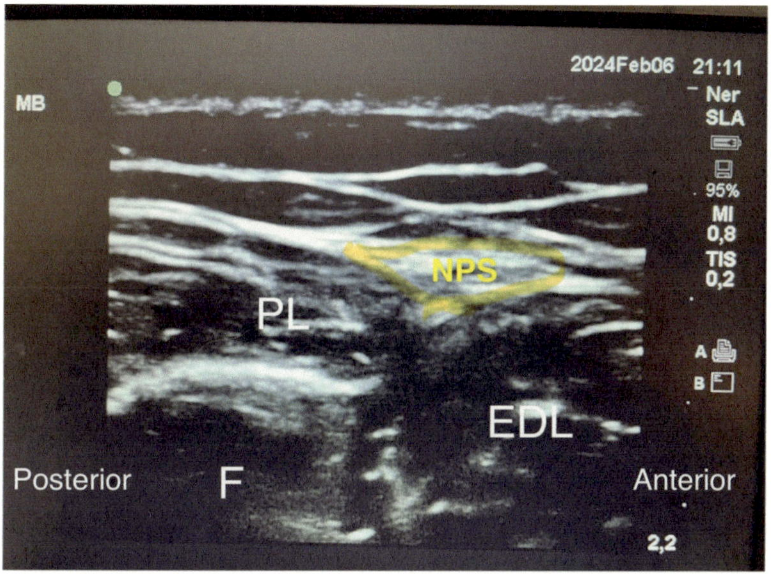

Figure 12.
Sonography of the superficial peroneal (fibula) nerve (NPS) at the distal third of the leg. The NPS is seen in the intermuscular septum between peroneus longus (PL) and extensor digitorum longus (EDL) deep to the crural fascia. Source: Authors.

the groove between the lower fibula (lateral malleolus) and the Achilles tendon (**Figure 13**), applying minimal pressure to prevent compression of the lesser saphenous vein. Both the vein and the nerve are situated within the fascial plane between the peroneus tendon and Achilles tendon (**Figure 14**). The sural nerve is observed as a small, round hyperechoic structure located adjacent to the lesser saphenous vein

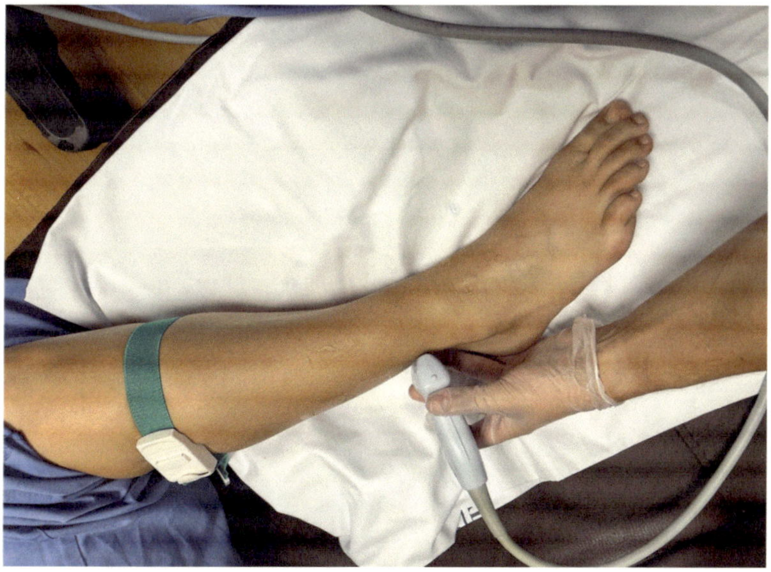

Figure 13.
Patient position and transducer for sural nerve block. Source: Authors.

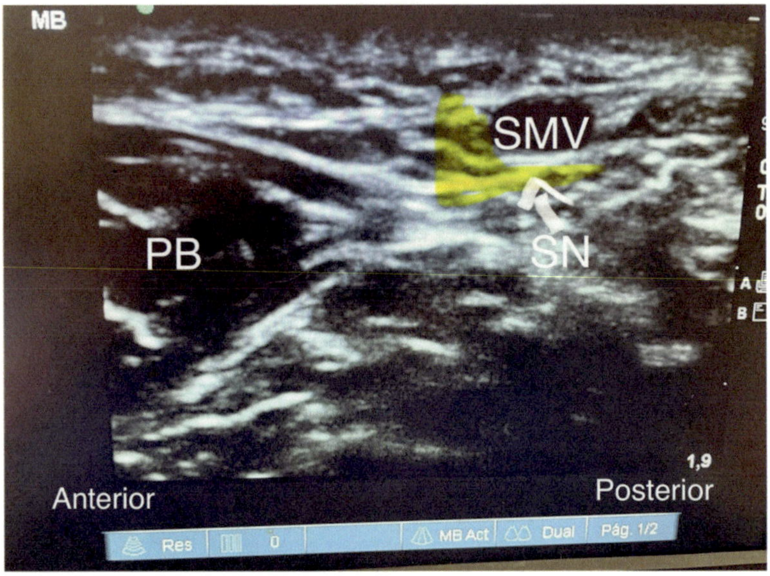

Figure 14.
Sonography of the sural nerve (indicated by line arrow). It is accompanied by the lesser saphenous vein, and both are located within the fascia plane (block arrows) between the peroneus brevis (PB) muscle and tendon Achilles (TA). Source: Author.

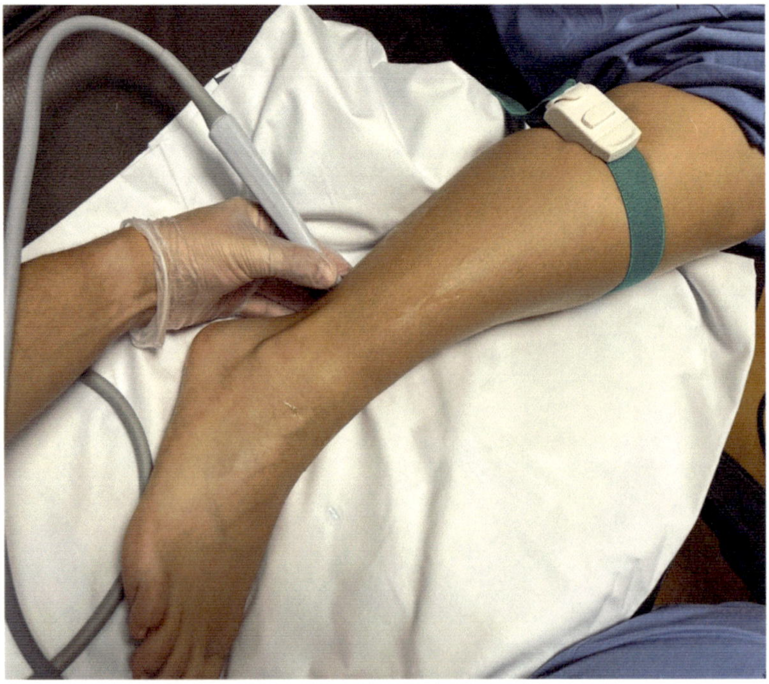

Figure 15.
A tourniquet can be placed around the calf to enhance the venous filling. Source: Author.

within the same fascial subcutaneous plane. If the sural nerve is not immediately visible, the peroneal sheath can be located, with the nerve typically found anteriorly and outside it. Another method to aid in visualizing the sural nerve is to apply a tourniquet to the upper third of the leg to distend the small saphenous vein and facilitate locating the nerve (as shown in **Figure 15**) [30, 43].

The target for injection is the fascial expansion between the fibula and Achilles tendon. If the nerve remains elusive, local anesthetic can be injected around the vein. The nerve may be approached using either an in-plane or out-of-plane technique, with caution taken to avoid piercing the nerve itself. A volume of 3–5 ml of local anesthetic is then injected into the fascial plane surrounding the nerve.

In a study by Redborg et al. [43], a randomized, prospective, and blinded study was conducted with 18 healthy volunteers divided into two groups: one receiving sural nerve block guided by ultrasound and the other by anatomical landmarks. The study concluded that ultrasound-guided (USG) techniques produced a more comprehensive and longer-lasting block.

6. Conclusion

With the development of US we are enabled to perform very selective and precise nerve blocks. The primary clinical justification for employing ultrasound guidance lies in its capacity to pinpoint the precise location of the nerve, offer real-time visualization of the needle, and allow observation of the spread of local anesthetic, providing immediate feedback to the practitioner [44].

One of the best examples of the accuracy of this technology is the ankle block, small sensory end nerves, at the ankle level, can be identified and blocked using very low dose comparing with landmark techniques.

The ankle block is an effective regional technique, providing excellent intraoperative anesthesia as well as long postoperative pain relief in foot surgeries, the advantages are less motor block with similar analgesic effectiveness compared to sciatic block [45]. In the context of modern times, this holds greater significance in outpatient scenarios due to the implementation of enhanced recovery programs and fast-track orthopedic surgery protocols, which prioritize rapid patient mobility and discharge [9]. Some evidence suggests that the USG technique improves block success rates, facilitates faster block progression, without prolonging the procedure time [46].

7. Practical tips

- When administering the ankle block, prioritize blocking the tibial nerve first, as it is the largest nerve and takes longer to achieve a full block onset [24].

- During the superficial peroneal nerve block, begin scanning from a higher position when the nerve is deep to the crural fascia, and observe its emergence superficially. The nerve may be challenging to visualize in this location due to its smaller size and hypoechoic nature [24].

- Visualizing the deep peroneal and saphenous nerves can pose challenges. However, by concentrating on the fascial plane that delineates the vessel, inject the local anesthetic within that plane. The sural nerve consistently resides within the fascial expansion between the peroneus and Achilles tendons [24].

- Patients undergoing this block should be adequately sedated since it involves multiple needle insertions and superficial injections of local anesthetic, which can cause discomfort. Patient alertness is not crucial for the block [28].

- When injecting local anesthetic to block superficial nerves, ensure the presence of a wheal to confirm correct placement of the needle in the superficial plane [28].

- Both the posterior tibial and deep peroneal nerves are situated deep to the fascia [28].

- Ankle block used for outpatient foot surgery enables most patients to walk with assistance, facilitating earlier discharge from the surgical center [28].

Author details

Alberto De La Espriella
Department of Anesthesia, Hospital Universitario San Ignacio, Bogota, Colombia

*Address all correspondence to: adespriella@husi.org.co

References

[1] Collins L, Halwani A, Vaghadia H. Impact of a regional anesthesia analgesia program for outpatient foot surgery. Canadian Journal of Anaesthesia. 1999;**46**:840-845

[2] Chelly JE, Greger J, Casati A, Al-Samsam T, McGarvey W, Clanton T. Continuous lateral sciatic blocks for acute postoperative pain management after major ankle and foot surgery. Foot & Ankle International. 2002;**23**:749-752

[3] Pearce CJ, Hamilton PD. Current concepts review: Regional anesthesia for foot and ankle surgery. Foot & Ankle International. 2010;**31**:732-739

[4] Stefani KC, Ferreira GF, Pereira Filho MV. Postoperative analgesia using peripheral anesthetic block of the foot and ankle. Foot & Ankle International. 2018;**39**:196-200

[5] Chaudier P, Bourdin M, Gauthier J, et al. Similar levels of pain are reported in forefoot surgery after management as a day case and admission for 48 hours: A continuous prospective study of 317 patients. The Bone and Joint Journal. 2015;**97-B**:1645-1650

[6] Mouton A, Le Strat V, Medevielle D, et al. Patient's satisfaction after outpatient forefoot surgery: Study of 619 cases. Orthopaedics & Traumatology, Surgery & Research. 2015;**101**:S217-S220

[7] Merrill HM, Dean DM, Mottla JL, et al. Opioid consumption following foot and ankle surgery. Foot & Ankle International. 2018;**39**:649-656

[8] Korwin-Kochanowska K, Potié A, El-Boghdadly K, Rawal N, Joshi G, Albrecht E. PROSPECT/ESRA Working Group Collaboration. PROSPECT guideline for hallux valgus repair surgery: a systematic review and procedure-specific postoperative pain management recommendations. Regional Anesthesia and Pain Medicine. Sep 2020;**45**(9):702-708. DOI: 10.1136/rapm-2020-101479. Epub 2020 Jun 28. PMID: 32595141; PMCID: PMC7476301

[9] Marty P, Rontes O, Chassery C, et al. Perineural versus systemic dexamethasone in front-foot surgery under ankle block: A randomized double-blind study. Regional Anesthesia and Pain Medicine. 2018;**43**:732-737

[10] Hofmann-Kiefer KF, Gaube F, Groene P, Böcker W, Polzer H, Baumbach SF. “High ankle block” for surgery at the ankle joint. Foot and Ankle Surgery. Dec 2022;**28**(8):1254-1258. DOI: 10.1016/j.fas.2022.05.006. Epub 2022 May 26. PMID: 35654730

[11] Delbos A, Philippe M, Clément C, Olivier R, Coppens S. Ultrasound-guided ankle block. History revisited. Best Practice & Research. Clinical Anaesthesiology. 2019;**33**(1):79-93. DOI: 10.1016/j.bpa.2019.05.002. PMID: 31272656. Epub 2019 May 7

[12] Fredrickson MJ. Ultrasound-guided ankle block. Anaesthesia and Intensive Care. 2009;**37**:143-144

[13] Bindu S, Mazumder S, Bandyopadhyay U. Non-steroidal anti-inflammatory drugs (NSAIDs) and organ damage: A current perspective. Biochemical Pharmacology. 2020;**180**:114147. DOI: 10.1016/j.bcp.2020.114147

[14] Burd TA, Hughes MS, Anglen JO. Heterotopic ossification prophylaxis with indomethacin increases the risk of long-bone nonunion. The Journal of

Bone and Joint Surgery. British Volume. 2003;**85**:700-705

[15] Chrastil J, Sampson C, Jones KB, Higgins TF. Postoperative opioid administration inhibits bone healing in an animal model. Clinical Orthopaedics and Related Research. 2013;**471**:4076-4081. DOI: 10.1007/s11999-013-3232-z

[16] Scuderi GR. The challenges of perioperative pain management in total joint arthroplasty. The American Journal of Orthopedics. 2015;**44**:S2-S4

[17] Fraser TW, Doty JF. Peripheral nerve blocks in foot and ankle surgery. The Orthopedic Clinics of North America. 2017;**48**:507-515. DOI: 10.1016/j.ocl.2017.06.008

[18] Vadivelu N, Kai AM, Maslin B, Kodumudi V, Antony S, Blume P. Role of regional anesthesia in foot and ankle surgery. Foot & Ankle Specialist. 2015;**8**:212-219

[19] Albaqami MS, Alqarni AA. Efficacy of regional anesthesia using ankle block in ankle and foot surgeries: A systematic review. European Review for Medical and Pharmacological Sciences. Jan 2022;**26**(2):471-484. DOI: 10.26355/eurrev_202201_27872. PMID: 35113423

[20] Tryba M. Ankle block: A safe and simple technique for foot surgery. Current Opinion in Anaesthesiology. 1997;**10**:361-365

[21] Lee TH, Wapner KL, Hecht PJ, Hunt PJ. Regional anesthesia in foot and ankle surgery. Orthopedics. 1996;**19**:577-580

[22] Rudkin GE, Micallef TA. Impediments to the use of ankle block in Australia. Anaesthesia and Intensive Care. 2004;**32**:368-371

[23] López AM, Sala-Blanch X, Magaldi M, Poggio D, Asuncion J, Franco CD. Ultrasound-guided ankle block for forefootsurgery: The contribution of the saphenous nerve. Regional Anesthesia & Pain Medicine. 2012;**37**:554-557

[24] Peng P. Ankle nerve block. In: Jankovic D, Peng P, editors. Regional Nerve Blocks in Anesthesia and Pain Therapy. Cham: Springer; 2022. DOI: 10.1007/978-3-030-88727-8_67

[25] Hancock KJ, Rice OM, Anthony CA, Glass N, Hogue M, Karam M, et al. Efficacy of multimodal analgesic injections in operatively treated ankle fractures: A randomized controlled trial. The Journal of Bone and Joint Surgery. American Volume. 2019;**101**:2194-2202. DOI: 10.2106/jbjs.19.00293

[26] Davidovitch R, Goch A, Driesman A, Konda S, Pean C, Egol K. The use of liposomal bupivacaine administered with standard bupivacaine in ankle fractures requiring open reduction internal fixation: A single-blinded randomized controlled trial. Journal of Orthopaedic Trauma. 2017;**31**:434-439. DOI: 10.1097/bot.0000000000000862

[27] Kaller P, Hohenberger G, Holweg P, Seibert FJ, Ornig M. Ankle block. Operative Orthopädie und Traumatologie. 2020;**32**:29-34. DOI: 10.1007/s00064-019-00634-x

[28] Yared M, Brown DL. Ankle block. In: Brown's Atlas of Regional Anesthesia. 6th ed. Elsevier; 2021. pp. 157.e1-164.e1. ISBN: 978-0-323-65435-7

[29] Chin KJ, Wong NWY, Macfarlane AJR, Chan VWS. Ultrasound-guided versus anatomic landmark-guided ankle blocks: A 6-year retrospective review. Regional Anesthesia and Pain Medicine. 2011;**36**:611-618

[30] Girón-Arango L, Vásquez-Sadder MI, González-Obregón MP,

Gamero-Fajardo CE. Bloqueo de tobillo guiado por ultrasonido: Una técnica anestésica atractiva para cirugía de pie. Colombian Journal of Anesthesiology. 2015;**43**(4):283-289. Retrieved January 24, 2024, from http://www.scielo.org.co/scielo.php?script=sci_arttext&pid=S0120-33472015000400005&lng=en&tlng=es

[31] Peer S, Gruber H. Atlas of Peripheral Nerve Ultrasound. Berlin: Springer; 2013

[32] Delbos. Peripheral Nerve Blocks on DVD Version 3- Lower Limbs. Philadelphia: Lippincott; 2012

[33] Lawrence SJ. The deep peroneal nerve in the foot and ankle: An anatomic study. Foot & Ankle International. 1995;**16**:724-728

[34] Mazzella NL, McMillan AM. Contribution of the sural nerve to postural stability and cutaneous sensation of the lower limb. Foot & Ankle International. 2015;**36**:450-456

[35] Chen J, Lesser J, Hadzic A, Resta-Flarer F. The importance of the proximal saphenous nerve block for foot and ankle surgery. Regional Anesthesia and Pain Medicine. 2013;**38**:372

[36] Fredrickson MJ, White R, Danesh-Clough TK. Low-volume ultrasound-guided nerve block provides inferior postoperative analgesia compared to a higher-volume landmark technique. Regional Anesthesia and Pain Medicine. 2011;**36**:393-398

[37] Lin E, Gaur A, Jones M, Ahmed A. Sonoanatomy for Anesthetists. United Kingdom: Cambridge University Press; 2012

[38] Redborg KE, Antonakakis JG, Beach ML, Chinn CD, Sites BD. Ultrasound improves the success rate of a tibial nerve block at the ankle. Regional Anesthesia and Pain Medicine. 2009;**34**:256-260

[39] De Mey JC, Deruyck LJ, Cammu G, de Baerdemaeker LE, Mortier EP. A paravenous approach for the saphenous nerve block. Regional Anesthesia and Pain Medicine. 2001;**26**:504-550

[40] Antonakakis J, Scalzo DC, Jorgenson AS, Figg KK, Ting P, Zuo Z, et al. Ultrasound does not improve the success rate of a deep peroneal nerve block at the ankle. Regional Anesthesia and Pain Medicine. 2010;**35**:217-221

[41] Canella C, Demondion X, Guillin R, Boutry N, Peltier J, Cotten A. Anatomic study of the superficial peroneal nerve using sonography. AJR. American Journal of Roentgenology. 2009;**193**:174-179

[42] Chin KJ. Ultrasound visualization of the superficial peroneal nerve in the mid-calf. Anesthesiology. 2013;**118**:956-965

[43] Redborg KE, Sites BD, Chinn CD, Gallagher JD, Ball PA, Antonakakis JG, et al. Ultrasound improves the success rate of a sural nerve block at the ankle. Regional Anesthesia and Pain Medicine. 2009;**34**:24-28

[44] Falyar CR. Ultrasound-guided ankle blocks: A review of current practices. AANA Journal. 2015;**83**:357-364

[45] Migues A, Slullitel G, Vescovo A, DroblasF,CarrascoM,PerrinTH.Peripheral foot blockade versus popliteal fossa nerve block: A prospective randomized trial in 51 patients. The Journal of Foot and Ankle Surgery. 2005;**44**:354-357

[46] Gbejuade H, Squire J, Dixit A, Kaushik V, Mangwani J. Ultrasound-guided regional anesthesia in foot and ankle surgery. Journal of Clinical Orthopaedics and Trauma. 2020;**11**:417-421

Chapter 4

Severe Traumatic Brain Injury: Acute Treatment Based on Cerebral Perfusion Pressure

Theno Alexandro Turrubiates Hernández, Gabriela María Mora Martínez, Amalia Angélica Reyes Pérez, Ramón Ulises Soberano Burguete, Gustavo Adrián Soto Hernandez, Brenda Lizbeth González Zúñiga and Rodolfo Antonio Valerio Aguirre

Abstract

Severe traumatic brain injury is a cause of disability with economic and social repercussions. Prehospital care is a fundamental part with important attention to avoid hypoxemia, hyperventilation, and hypotension with airway protection. During the primary evaluation, a clinical examination is performed focused on classifying according to their severity, neurological involvement, and extracranial lesions and providing a prognosis. Invasive or non-invasive intracranial pressure monitoring aims to direct management to maintain adequate cerebral perfusion pressure, which should be individualized in each patient, as this depends on the status of self-regulation.

Keywords: traumatic brain injury, cerebral perfusion pressure, intracranial pressure, intracranial hypertension, trauma

1. Introduction

Traumatic brain injury (TBI) is defined as an injury to brain caused by an external force on the head that can be a blow, explosion, or penetrating injury [1]. It causes severe disability among young people with economic and social repercussions. Existing limitations to treatment in underdeveloped countries include inadequate prehospital care, limited advanced neuromonitoring techniques, or availability of intensive care [2, 3].

Globally, it is estimated that in 2016, there were 55 million patients diagnosed with TBI, the annual cost of the likely economic losses of productivity was $1.2 billion [4]. Approximately, 69 million people each year are affected by this clinical entity, it should be noted that in this study, it showed a threefold higher incidence in developing countries [5].

In the United States, around 1.7 million people are diagnosed with TBI per year, with the most affected population being between 15 and 19 years of age, as well as those over 65 years of age, with a 2:1 ratio with a predominance of males [6]. The mortality associated with a closed traumatic injury grows exponentially when it is associated with a brain injury, which is why prehospital rapid response emergency teams play an important role [7].

Prehospital care is a fundamental part of reducing complications in patients with TBI, there are three important pillars in prehospital care, which are avoiding hypoxemia (maintaining a saturation greater than 94%), protecting the airway by evaluating the need for endotracheal intubation, and avoiding hyperventilation and hypotension [7, 8].

TBIs accounted for approximately 2.5 million emergency department visits in the United States, of which 87% (2,213,826) were treated and discharged from the emergency room; The other 11% (283,630) were admitted to hospitalization and were discharged in the following days, and approximately 2% (52,844) died in the hospital [9]. On the other hand, this pathology has significant effects on the quality of life of those people who suffer from this disease, it is estimated that in the United States, there are 3.2 to 5.3 million people living with a disability related to TBI [10].

There is evidence that patients with moderate to severe TBI who were discharged from rehabilitation were more than twice as likely to die after 3 to 5 years compared to people in the general population who were the same age, sex, and race [11].

2. Brain physiology

2.1 Brain metabolism

The human brain weighs approximately 1350 grams, which represents 2% of the total weight of an adult [12]. It takes up more energy than any other organ. Glucose is the main source of brain energy; It does not freely diffuse the blood-brain barrier. It enters the brain by active transport via glucose transporter (GLUT) 1, it is distributed to the central nervous system by several transporters (GLUT 1, GLUT 3, GLUT 5). These transporters undergo regulation with a tendency to rise under certain conditions, such as hypoxia [13].

The generation of brain energy under conditions of oxygen and glucose at normal levels is carried out by means of glycolysis by oxidative phosphorylation of creatine phosphokinase and adenylyl cyclase. The process allows the formation of 3 molecules of adenosine triphosphate (ATP) for each nicotinamide adenine dinucleotide (NADH) and a maximum of 38 molecules of ATP is obtained for each molecule of glucose. In the absence of oxygen in astrocytes, anaerobic glucose metabolism is performed to form lactate and ATP is generated to capture glutamate. Lactate is taken up by neurons and transformed into pyruvate that initiates the citric acid cycle, in this process, hydrogen ions are released which are associated with acidosis and more brain damage. In this way, ATP generation is lower per glucose molecule, generating only 2 ATP molecules per glucose molecule, which is not enough for brain demands [13].

On the other hand, during a prolonged fast, the brain uses ketone bodies which are broken down into acetyl coenzyme A to be oxidized in the citric acid cycle, so in extreme conditions, the brain can produce low amounts of energy from gluconeogenesis using glycerol, glutamine, and glycine as substrates. With low oxygen levels, ATP generation then drops and phosphocreatine deposits are occupied until anaerobic metabolism is exhausted, resulting in the cessation of electrical activity in the brain. Maintaining normal blood glucose levels is essential for normal brain function. The brain is particularly sensitive to hypoglycemia because there are no glycogen stores [14].

2.2 Cerebral circulation

The cerebral irrigation is given by the internal carotid arteries, which branch and give rise to the anterior circulation, the vertebral arteries give rise to the basilar artery and its branches give rise to the posterior circulation [15].

The brain occupies approximately 15% of cardiac output (750 ml/min) and maintains a cerebral blood flow of 50 ml/100 g/minute. In the resting state, the brain consumes oxygen at an approximate rate of 3.5 ml/100 g/minute, which represents 20% of the body's total consumption [16].

Cerebral perfusion pressure (CPP) is defined as the difference between mean arterial pressure (MAP) and intracranial pressure (ICP). Under normal conditions in adults, it ranges between 60 and 150 mmHg and the ICP around 10 mmHg [16].

2.3 Monro-Kellie theory

The skull, after the closure of the sutures and fontanelles, becomes an inextensible configuration and, therefore, maintains a constant volume regardless of the contents. Under normal conditions, this content can be separated into three components (Monro-Kellie's theory): brain 80%, cerebrospinal fluid (CSF) 10%, and blood 10%, respectively. When there is an increase in the volume of any of the three components, the pressure exerted by that component on the other two also increases. The CSF is the main compensatory system [15].

2.4 Partial pressure of carbon dioxide (PaCO2) and its implication in cerebral blood flow

The acid-base state and its regulation have been shown to have a direct effect on cerebral blood flow (CBF), causing a series of changes that have implications for health, for years, it has been an important area of study in which CBF, PaCO2, bicarbonate (HCO-3), and pH are integrated.

The cerebral circulation varies with the levels of PaCO2, in normal situations, the CBF increases from 2 to 4% of mmHg with an increase of PaCO2, making P toCO2 the most potent physiological vasodilator [17].

The response seen in CBF to changes from PaCO2 occurs in seconds and completes equilibrium within 1 to 2 minutes due to rapid diffusion across the blood-brain barrier (BBB) to perivascular fluid and cerebral vascular smooth muscle cells.

Changes in CBF secondary to PaCO2 levels are not sustained for prolonged periods. The adaptation point in the pH of CBF is observed at 6 hours with subsequent decrease in secondary changes to PaCO2 [12, 18].

3. Clinical classifications for TBI

The primary evaluation of a patient with TBI consists of a clinical examination focused on classifying according to its severity, neurological, and even structural involvement, as well as providing prognosis.

The Glasgow Coma Scale (GCS) (score from 3 to 15 pts) and the FOUR scale (score from 0 to 16 pts) are among the most commonly used scales to assess and identify the patient's state of consciousness and guide management [19, 20].

It is recommended to establish a single scale for the progressive evaluation of the patient at 6, 12, 24, and 72 hours of the patient and to avoid marked differences in the patient's approach and prognosis [21–23].

3.1 Tomographic classification

Computed tomography (CT) classifications of TBI lesions are used to establish prognosis, estimate risks of intracranial hypertension (IH), and thus establish probable surgical treatment. The most commonly used classifications for these types of scenarios are Marshall and Rotterdam. Other classifications, such as Helsinki and Stockholm, have demonstrated good sensitivity and specificity in some studies for predicting decline, but it still does not exceed the previous ones mentioned in use [24].

3.1.1 Marshall's tomographic classification

Standard method for the evaluation of CT in traumatic brain injury involves evaluating the mesencephalic cisterns, midline, presence or absence of hemorrhage and whether or not they were evacuated, as well as cerebral edema, generating a percentage risk of IH and mortality or poor clinical outcomes. Mortality and the risk of IH increase with each grade of the scale, up to 55 and 63% respectively in grade III and 100% in grade IV. In addition to these degrees, two more are described that refer to whether these hemorrhagic masses were evacuated or not; in the case of the evacuated mass, the mortality has been described between 33 and 52% and in the non-evacuated, the mortality reaches up to 80% [25, 26].

3.1.2 Rotterdam tomographic scale

A scale that values epidural hematoma and subarachnoid hemorrhage, demonstrating better performance than the Marshall classification for the 6-month prognosis, with similar results in terms of mortality. But the fact of individualizing the lesions gives you a better picture of exploration and quantification of risk. In scores 1 and 2, the mortality is 0%, in score 3, the mortality is up to 6%, in score 4, the mortality is 35%, in score 5, the mortality percentage is 54%, and in score 6, the mortality reaches 60% [25–27].

4. Neuromonitoring in the emergency room

Neuromonitoring encompasses direct and indirect techniques that help to provide early evidence of neuraxial damage and focus on reducing secondary injury by optimizing the balance between oxygen consumption and demand [28, 29]. Invasive and non-invasive surrogate PCI monitoring techniques and measurements will be addressed as a treatment guide in the emergency department.

4.1 Neurological monitoring strategies in the emergency room

4.1.1 Clinical neurological examination

The mainstay of clinical assessment is state of consciousness, such as GCS and FOUR [30, 31]. These scales should be complemented by an assessment of pupillary, cranial nerves, mobility, sensation, and limb strength.

4.1.2 Computed tomography

CT scan is the most widely used study to assess changes in the brain and can provide qualitative information on the increase in PCI [32]. It is preferred for its availability, speed, low cost, and ease of use in patients under mechanical ventilation [33].

4.2 Non-invasive intracranial pressure monitoring

4.2.1 Transcranial Doppler (TCD)

In the initial evaluation of patients with severe TBI, TCD measurements may help guide treatment and decrease mortality [34].

TCD is a non-invasive ultrasound that uses a low-frequency transducer (<2 MHz) that detects the intracranial circulation through an acoustic bony window, is based on emissions and flow receptions, the angle and position of the insonation must be adjusted to provide the best Doppler signal [35, 36].

The acoustic windows used are transorbital, temporal, submandibular, and foramen magnum. In clinical practice, the middle cerebral artery (MCA) is the most insonable due to its easy access through the temporal window above the zygomatic arch, it has a sensitivity of 38–91%, specificity of 94–100% prediction of vasospasm [37]. The TCD measures flow rates, spectral wave analysis, and various indices that vary according to the insonation window and the vessel analyzed.

- The pulsatibility index (PI) is calculated as:

$$PI = Peak\ systolic\ flow - Peak\ diastolic\ flow \div Mean\ velocity \tag{1}$$

The normal value of PI is between 0.6 and 1.16, a PI less than 0.6 is associated with vasospasm, hyperemia, or high-grade stenosis; a PI between 1.2 and 1.6 is associated with moderate IH or microangiopathy, a PI greater than 1.7–3 with severe IH, and values greater than 3 are associated with severe IH and cerebral asystole [37]. The PCI can be estimated based on the PI with the following equation [38]:

$$ICP = (10.927\ X\ PI - 1.284) + / - 3.2 - 12\ mmHg \tag{2}$$

- The Resistance Index (RI) which is calculated as:

$$RI = \frac{peak\ systolic\ flow - peak\ diastolic\ flow}{peak\ systolic\ flow} \tag{3}$$

It increases in the early stages of IH and in old age [16]. Anything per <0.75 is considered normal [39].

- Lindegaard Index (LI)

It is a value that normalizes the flow velocity of the AMC with respect to internal carotid arteries (ICA), it serves to differentiate hyperemia from true vasospasm. A normal LI is considered <3, mild vasospasm 3.0–4.5, moderate 4.5–6.0, and severe >6.0 [39]. It is calculated as:

$$LI = \frac{Flow\ velocity\ of\ CMA}{Flow\ velocity\ of\ ACI} \tag{4}$$

4.2.2 Optic nerve sheath diameter (ONSD)

The optic nerve is an extension of the central nervous system, lined by meninges and cerebrospinal fluid (**Figure 1**). The optic nerve sheath (ONS) is in continuity with the meninges, specifically the dura mater. It is the intraorbital segment of the optic nerve and is separated from it by cerebrospinal fluid and the arachnoid trabeculae [1, 4]. The elevation of the PCI causes the CSF to be distributed through the dura mater toward the ONS, increasing its diameter [40].

Several studies have validated the linear relationship between the measurement of ONS by ultrasound with invasive methods and PCI, with detection of ICP elevation

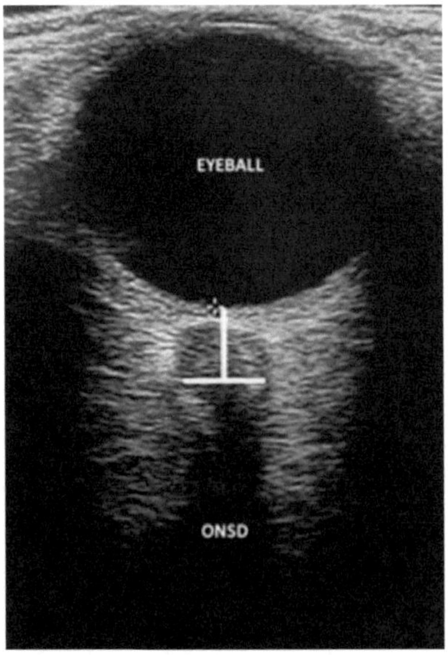

Figure 1.
ONSD measurement. Optic nerve sheath diameter (ONSD).

in ranges of 4.8–5.6 mm with an overall sensitivity and specificity of 95 and 92%, respectively [41].

Serial measurement of the ONSD and the use of the following validated formula for inference of PCI with the ONSD [42] are recommended:

$$ICP = (ONSD\ in\ mm\ x\ 5.69) - 8.23 \tag{5}$$

This method should not be used in patients with facial trauma, Graves' disease, and sarcoidosis [31].

ONSD measurement is a validated non-invasive method that is easy and quick to use. Performing it together with DCT in patients with severe TBI upon admission to the emergency room can be taken as a guide for initiation of treatment and neuroprotective measures [43].

4.2.3 Other methods

Near-infrared spectroscopy (NIRS) has an uncertain sensitivity for recognizing increased PCI, yet it is considered a complementary non-invasive method in neurological monitoring, limited by its non-specificity and restricted availability [44]. Another method, such as quantitative optical pupillometry, may be useful to guide response to osmotic treatment or as a monitoring of PCI, but its use in emergency departments has not been reported [45].

4.2.4 Continuous electroencephalogram (cEEG)

cEEG provides neuronal information in response to changes in brain structure or function. It is a continuous registry, fast and easy to use, however, with a high cost. It is used for the detection of non-convulsive status epilepticus and cerebral ischemia (CBF < 25–35 mL/100 g/min, alpha and beta waves are attenuated, and if CBF <17–18 mL/100 g/min, slow delta and zeta waves are increased) [46].

4.3 Invasive intracranial pressure monitoring in the emergency room

4.3.1 Jugular bulb saturation (SjvO2)

It is a minimally invasive method of neuromonitoring. Currently, an ultrasound-guided fiber optic catheter is placed, both sides can be catheterized, however, right placement is more common [47].

SjvO2 measures the relationship between brain metabolic requirements and blood flow, being a direct determination of brain oxygen consumption (CMRO2) [48, 49].

It has a normal value of 55 to 75%, a low SjvO2 is associated with vasospasm, ischemia, or metabolic cause (fever, chills, agitation). Elevated SjvO2 is associated with hyperemia, hyperoxia, arteriovenous shunt, or extensive cerebral infarction. Although it is part of the monitoring in TBI guidelines, it is rarely used in the emergency department [49].

4.3.2 External ventricular drainage

External ventricular drainage (EVD) is globally considered the gold standard for PCI monitoring. It is used as continuous monitoring of PCI and treatment of IH for

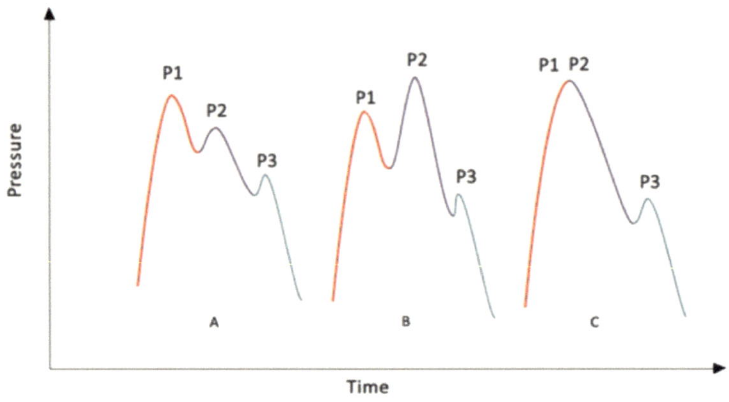

Figure 2.
Morphology of ICP waves. (A) Normal ICP curve. (B) Decreased cerebral compliance with increased P2. (C) Decreased compliance with critical increase in ICP. Intracranial pressure (ICP).

various pathologies (acute hydrocephalus, hematomas, hemorrhages, severe TBI, tumor, infection, or cerebral edema) [50]. It is associated with complications such as obstruction, improper placement, infections, and bleeding [51].

The components of the ICP wave are:

- P1 is the arterial component (percussive wave). It originates from the pulsation of the choroid plexus, it has constant amplitude.
- P2 represents intracranial compliance (tidal wave).
- P3 is associated with the closure of the aortic valve (dicrotic wave).

P2 and P3 are produced from the retrograde venous beat of the jugular veins over cortical veins, between which the dicrote cleft of the pulse occurs. The change in the P2 wave is indicative of IH and consequently loss of brain self-regulation (**Figure 2**) [52].

5. Treatment of severe TBI

The presence of other extracranial lesions should be considered in the management of patients with severe TBI. Post-traumatic bleeding is one of the most common causes of death in patients with TBI associated with other injuries, and is a preventable cause of death [53, 54]. Therefore, priority should be given to controlling bleeding in case of hemodynamic instability, considering medical and surgical management [54].

It is recommended that during bleeding control, a hemoglobin (Hb) greater than 7 g/dL and, in some cases, higher levels be maintained, for example, in patients with low myocardial reserve or previous heart disease and older adults. If surgical management is warranted, a platelet count greater than 50,000/mm^3 and an INR of less than 1.5 should be maintained. A partial pressure oxygen (PaO2) level of 60 to 100 mmHg and a PaCO2 of 35 to 40 mmHg are maintained to ensure adequate oxygen transport [54, 55].

In hemodynamic control, a MAP greater than 80 mmHg or a systolic blood pressure (SBP) greater than 100 mmHg is sought, in case these pressure levels make it difficult to control bleeding, lower levels could be considered for short periods [55]. In addition, during the management of bleeding, consider massive transfusion protocols, as well as the use of thromboelastography (TEG) and rotational thromboelastometry (ROTEM) to guide the decision to use blood products [56].

After hemorrhage control, the severity of the brain injury should be assessed by means of pupillary evaluation, the level of consciousness with the GCS, and the performance of an imaging study [57, 58].

When performing the tomographic study, the presence of potentially surgical life-threatening intracranial lesions should be sought, and in such a case, an emergency evaluation by the neurosurgeon should be requested, who will regulate surgical management [59].

Within the management of PCI, the factors that are related to worse outcomes are values greater than 20 to 25 mmHg and the duration of the outcomes [58, 60]. The goal of management is to maintain an adequate PPC, which must be individualized in each patient, since this depends on the status of self-regulation [61], therapy should not only focus on maintaining a specific value in all patients. It is suggested in most guidelines and studies that maintaining a PPC value between 60 and 70 mmHg has better outcomes and fewer neurological sequelae [62]. PPC values above 100 mmHg are related to vasogenic edema and values below 50 mmHg are related to cerebral ischemia [61, 63].

Among the measures that can reduce PCI in order to improve PPC are osmotherapy (20% mannitol or hypertonic saline), external interventricular drainage, and hyperventilation [4, 6]. Patients with IH such as respiratory depression, bradycardia, hypertension, or signs of cerebral herniation (mydriasis or anisocoria) require immediate medical treatment with one of these options. Prophylactic use in the absence of data on increased PCI with osmotherapy over conventional therapy has not shown improvement in outcomes [62].

Mannitol and hypertonic saline (**Table 1**) are similar in efficacy in the control of IH [64, 65]. The decision of which osmotic therapy to use should be based on consideration of its adverse effects and the clinical scenario, as in the case of mannitol that generates osmotic diuresis and hypovolemia, which would have to be made

	Bolus dose	Mechanism of action	Disadvantages
Mannitol 20%	0.25 to 1 g/kg	• Reduces ICP due to osmotic effect at the brain level plus osmotic diuresis.	• Hyperosmolar hypovolemia • Risk of acute tubular necrosis • Hydroelectric alterations
Hypertonic solutions: 3% NaCl 5% NaCl 7.5% NaCl 10% NaCl 14.6% NaCl 23.4% NaCl	250 mL or 2.5–5 mL/kg 100 mL 2–4 mL/kg or 100 mL 75 mL 24–48 mL 30 mL (0.686–2.0 mL/kg)	• Increase in intravascular volume. • Osmotic gradient decreasing brain volume. • Improved rheology of the blood.	• Risk of hyperchloremic acidosis • Risk of pontine myelinolysis • Electrolyte disorders

Table 1.
Characteristics of the osmotherapy. Abbreviations: Sodium chloride (NaCl).

in conjunction with volume expansion to avoid undesirable hemodynamic effects. Hypertonic saline could be considered a better option in cases of hypovolemia due to the volume expansion it generates, however, both therapies warrant monitoring of serum sodium levels and water balances [65, 66].

The use of hyperventilation (PaCO2 25 to 30 mmHg) is effective for the management of IH, it is considered a transient therapy in which a definitive surgical management is carried out and in cases of imminent herniation. Prolonged use of hyperventilation has deleterious effects, as well as the risk of cerebral ischemia, due to its effects on cerebral vasculature [66, 67].

The use of antiepileptic drugs prophylactically for post-traumatic seizures is not routinely recommended [68]; their use is considered only in patients with risk factors, such as skull fracture, acute subdural hematoma, initial loss of consciousness, amnesia for more than 24 hours, and age greater than 65 years [68, 69].

Other therapies for the management of TBI can be mentioned, however, there is no evidence of benefit, such as the use of high doses of glucocorticoids or the use of albumin during fluid resuscitation; In both cases, an increase in mortality was observed when compared to conventional therapy [70, 71].

Within ventilatory management, the indication for orointubation and use of mechanical ventilation depends on a combination of factors ranging from the level of consciousness (GCS less than 8 pts), loss of airway protection reflexes, severe agitation, combative state, and significant elevation of PCI [72]. Regarding the scheduling of mechanical ventilation in patients with or without IH, the parameters may be similar to those of patients without TBI, maintaining a protective ventilation strategy (tidal volume 6 to 8 mL per predicted weight, PEEP 5 cmH2O, plateau pressure less than 30 cmH2O, and a respiratory rate of 16 to 22 breaths/minute) [73].

Ventilatory management can be staggered in the case of acute respiratory failure syndrome (ARDS), with an initial protective schedule with subsequent adjustments to avoid severe hypoxemia; The tidal volume will be adjusted to maintain a conduction pressure of less than 14 cmH2O, as well as the respiratory rate for controlled hypocapnia (PaCO2 of 32 to 35 mmHG) [74].

In case of worsening of ARDS, advanced strategies such as prone position and neuromuscular blockade should be considered in conjunction with osmotherapy with optimal MAP to ensure adequate PPC [74, 75].

Every patient with severe TBI should be given measures to maintain adequate homeostasis (keep the brain happy) [62]. Multiple mnemonics have been described to ensure measures that improve and ensure cerebral oxygenation in patients with TBI.

The mnemonics of THE MANTLE (**Table 2**) are used at the bedside of patients with severe TBI [76]. In the following paragraphs, we will describe what is suggested to evaluate in this mnemonic.

It is considered essential to avoid hyperthermia in these patients, this generates an increase in brain metabolism, and therefore risk of cerebral hypoxia; A temperature target of 36 to 37°C is sought [76, 77].

Maintaining adequate oxygen transport is important. A Hb between 7 and 9 g/dL is suggested for adequate oxygen transport and to avoid hypoxia [76, 78].

Serum electrolyte values and acid-base status are important for brain homeostasis; serum sodium levels of 135 to 145 mEq/L and avoiding hypotonic solutions are important to maintain an adequate osmolar gradient; in the base acid, a pH of 7.35 to 7.45 is suggested to avoid modification of the Hb dissociation curve and alteration of oxygen delivery to tissues and organs [76].

THE MANTLE mnemonics		
Temperature	36–37.5°C	Hemoglobin
7–9 gr/dl	Electrolytes your acid-basic status	Na + 140–150 mEq/L pH: 7.35–7.45 p50 = 26–28 mmHg
Metabolism	Sedation and analgesia SvjO2 > 55%	Arterial blood pressure
SABP >100–110 mmHg	Nutrition and glucose	Glycemia 110–180 mg/dL
Target of oxygen	PaO2 80–120 mmHg SaO2 > 95%	Lung protective ventilation
Vt 6–10 ml/kg PBW RR to achieve PaCO2 35–45 mmHg PP < 14 DP < 13 cm H2O	Edema and ICP control	ICP < 22 mmHg CPP 55–70 mmHg ONSD <5.8 mm, PI <1.2 Serial CT scan

Abbreviations: Cerebral perfusion pressure (CPP); systolic arterial blood pressure (SABP); tidal volume (Vt); respiratory rate (RR); Plateau pressure (PP); driving pressure (DP); intracranial pressure (ICP); predicted body weight (PBW); oxygen pressure at half arterial oxygen pressure (p50); optic nerve sheath diameter (ONSD); pulsatility index (PI); Computed Tomography (CT).

Table 2.
The MANTLE mnemonics.

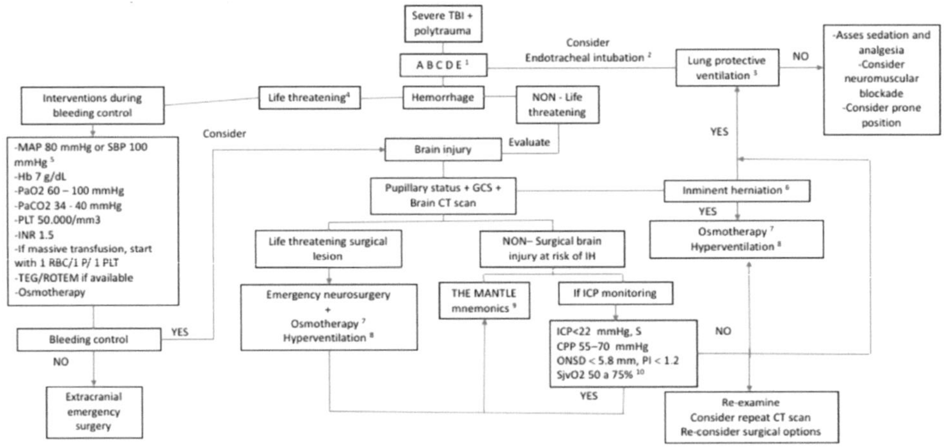

Figure 3.
Consensus algorithm. (1) primary assessment, (2) patient with impaired state of consciousness (GCS <8), (3) VT 6 to 8 ml, PEEP 5 cmH2O, PPLAT 30 cmH2O, RR of 16 to 22 breaths/minute, (4) bleeding with hemodynamic instability data, (5) in case of difficulty in controlling bleeding, consider lower values, (6) mydriasis or anisocoria, (7) mannitol or hypertonic saline, (8) maintain a PaCO2 of 25 to 30 mmHg, (9) follow mnemonics to maintain a happy brain, (10) consider maintaining adequate pain control, sedation, temperature, and agitation. Abbreviations: Tidal volume (VT), positive end-expiratory pressure (PEEP), plateau pressure (PPLAT), respiratory rate (RR), computed tomography (CT), Glasgow coma scale (GCS), mean arterial pressure (MAP), systolic blood pressure (SBP), hemoglobin (Hb), arterial partial pressure of oxygen (PaO2), arterial partial pressure of carbon dioxide (PaCO2), red blood cell (RBC), plasma (P), platelet (PLT), international normalized ratio (INR), thromboelastography (TEG), rotational thromboelastometry (ROTEM), intracranial pressure (ICP), cerebral perfusion pressure (CPP), intracranial hypertension (IH), optic nerve sheath diameter (ONSD), pulsatility index (PI), jugular bulb saturation (SjvO2).

Adequate sedation, pain control, agitation, and treatment of seizures are part of bedside assessment to prevent an increase in basal metabolic rate [76, 79].

As already mentioned, the avoidance of hypotension is of utmost importance, since it is related to worse outcomes, a BPS of 100 to 110 mmHg, maintaining a normal volume, a normal peripheral perfusion, a diuresis of at least 30 ml/hr., and a central venous pressure of 6 to 10 cmH2O are suggested [76, 80].

Glucose control is crucial for proper brain metabolism. A range of 110 to 180 mg/dL is suggested, since values outside this range are related to metabolic crises and generation of neurotoxic cascades that alter homeostasis [76, 81].

In terms of oxygenation, we have a PaO2 target of 80 to 110 mmHg and a SaO2 greater than 94%, avoiding hyperoxia as well as hypoxia [76]. In case of mechanical ventilation, pulmonary protection parameters should be maintained, as mentioned above [75, 76].

Finally, cerebral edema and PCI control should be given. In case of neurological monitoring, maintain a PCI of less than 22 mmHg, SjvO2 between 50 and 75%, and non-invasively, an ONSD <5.8 mm, a PI <1.2, and a brain computed tomography scan without signs of cerebral edema [76].

Within the management of patients with severe TBI, stepwise management is sought [82]. We recommend the algorithm in **Figure 3**, which is based on the recommendations previously discussed, always remembering the individualization of the patient.

6. Conclusion

The identification and appropriate approach of a patient with severe TBI, whether prehospital or Intra-hospital, requires a broad knowledge of brain physiology, in order to direct an appropriate neurological monitoring, whether invasive or non-invasive, and thus obtain information that allows us to direct a treatment in a staggered manner or controlling the ICP levels to guarantee the best CPP, taking into account variations in brain self-regulation. Regardless of the form in which the treatment is directed, the cornerstone is individualization.

Author details

Theno Alexandro Turrubiates Hernández[1*], Gabriela María Mora Martínez[2], Amalia Angélica Reyes Pérez[1], Ramón Ulises Soberano Burguete[1], Gustavo Adrián Soto Hernandez[1], Brenda Lizbeth González Zúñiga[3] and Rodolfo Antonio Valerio Aguirre[3]

1 Hospital Regional Cd Madero PEMEX, Mexico

2 Hospital de alta especialidad central sur PEMEX, Mexico

3 Hospital General Regional No 6 Cd Madero IMSS, Mexico

*Address all correspondence to: dr.turrubiates@outlook.es

References

[1] Hiskens M, Mengistus T, et al. Systematic review of the diagnostic and clinical utility of salivary micro RNAs in traumatic brain injury (TBI). International Journal of Molecular Sciences. 2022;**23**:13160. DOI: 10.3390/ijms232113160

[2] Rubiano AM, Griswold DP, Jibaja M, Rabinstein AA, Agustin GA. Management of severe traumatic brain injury in regions with limited resources. Brain Injury. 2021;**35**(11):1317-1325. DOI: 10.1080/02699052.2021.1972149

[3] Stein KY, Froese L, Gomez A, et al. Intracranial pressure monitoring and treatment thresholds in acute neural injury: A narrative review of the historical achievements, current state, and future perspectives. Neurotrauma Reports. 2023;**4**(1):478-494. DOI: 10.1089/neur.2023.0031

[4] Rolle ML, Garba DL, et al. The impact of traumatic brain injury on economic productivity in the Caribbean. Brain and Spine. 2023;**3**:101755. ISSN 2772-5294

[5] Joannides A, Korhonen TK, Clark D, et al. An international, prospective observational study on traumatic brain injury epidemiology study protocol: GEO-TBI: Incidence. NIHR Open Research. 2023;**3**:34. DOI: 10.3310/nihropenres.13377.1

[6] Georges A, Das M, J. Traumatic brain injury. In: StatPearls [Internet]. Treasure Island (FL): StatPearls Publishing; 2023

[7] Lulla A, Lumba-Brown A, et al. Prehospital guidelines for the management of traumatic brain injury – 3rd edition. Prehospital Emergency Care. 2023;**27**(5):507-538. DOI: 10.1080/10903127.2023.2187905

[8] Sun, Hai S, Navdeep S, et al. Impact of prehospital transportation on survival in skiers and snowboarders with traumatic brain injury. World Neurology. 2017;**104**:909-918.e8. DOI: 10.1016/j.wneu.2017.05.108

[9] Capizzi AN, Woo J, Verduzco-Gutierrez M. Traumatic brain injury. Medical Clinics of North America. 2020;**104**(2):213-238. DOI: 10.1016/j.mcna.2019.11.001

[10] Selassie AW et al. Incidence of long-term disability following traumatic brain injury hospitalization, United States. Journal of Head Trauma Rehabilitation. 2003;**23**(2):123-131. DOI: 10.1097/01.HTR.0000314531.30401.39

[11] Harrison-Felix C et al. Mortality after surviving traumatic brain injury risks based on age groups. Journal of Head Trauma Rehabilitation. 2012;**27**(6):E45-E56. DOI: 10.1097/HTR.0b013e31827340ba

[12] Vavilala MS, Lee LA, Lam AM. Cerebral blood flow and vascular physiology. Anesthesiology Clinics of North America. 2002;**20**(2):247-264. DOI: 10.1016/s0889-8537(01)00012-8

[13] Golding EM, Robertson CS, Bryan RM. The consequences of traumatic brain injury on cerebral blood flow and autoregulation: A review. Clinical and Experimental Hypertension. 1999;**21**(4):299-332. DOI: 10.3109/10641969909068668

[14] Taylor C, Hirsch N. Applied cerebral physiology. Anaesthesia & Intensive Care Medicine. 2007;**8**(10):407-412. DOI: 10.1016/j.mpaic.2007.08.010

[15] Stratmann G. Neurotoxicity of anesthetic drugs in the developing

brain. Anesthesia & Analgesia. 2011;**113**(5):1170-1179. DOI: 10.1213/ane.0b013e318232066c

[16] Avitsian R, Schubert A. Anesthetic considerations for intraoperative management of cerebrovascular disease in neuro-vascular surgical procedures. Anesthesiology Clinics. 2007;**25**:441-463. DOI: 10.1016/j.anclin.2007.06.002

[17] Caldwell HG, Carr JMJR, Minhas JS, Swenson ER, Ainslie PN. Acid-base balance and cerebrovascular regulation. The Journal of Physiology. 2021;**599**(24):5337-5359. DOI: 10.1113/jp281517

[18] Robinson C. Moderate and severe traumatic brain injury. Continuum: Lifelong Learning in Neurology. 2021;**27**(5):1278-1300. DOI: 10.1212/con.0000000000001036

[19] Mehta R, Trainee G, Chinthapalli K, Neurologist C. Glasgow coma scale explained. BMJ. 2019;**365**:l1296. DOI: 10.1136/bmj.l1296

[20] Barea-Mendoza JA, Llompart-Pou JA, Pérez-Bárcena J, Quintana-Díaz M, Serviá-Goixart L, Guerrero-López F, et al. External validation of the glasgow coma scale with pupillary assessment in patients with severe traumatic brain injury. Emergencies. 2023;**31**(1):34-45

[21] McNett M, Amato S, Philippbar SA. A comparative study of Glasgow coma scale and full outline of unresponsiveness scores for predicting long-term outcome after brain injury. Journal of Neuroscience Nursing. 2016;**48**(4):207-214. DOI: 10.1097/jnn.0000000000000225

[22] McNett M, Amato S, Gianakis A, Grimm D, Philippbar SA, Belle J, et al. The four score and GCS as predictors of outcome after traumatic brain injury. Neurocritical Care. 2014;**21**(1):52-57. DOI: 10.1007/s12028-013-9947-6

[23] Ghelichkhani P, Esmaeili M, Hosseini M, Seylani K. Glasgow coma scale and FOUR score in predicting the mortality of trauma patients; a diagnostic accuracy study. Emergency. 2018;**6**(1):1-7

[24] Thelin EP, Nelson DW, Vehviläinen J, Nyström H, Kivisaari R, Siironen J, et al. Evaluation of novel computerized tomography scoring systems in human traumatic brain injury: An observational, multicenter study. PLoS Medicine. 2017;**14**(8):e1002368. DOI: 10.1371/journal.pmed.1002368

[25] Ricardez-Cazares LG, González-Fernández MA, Dehesa-López E, Peraza-Garay F. Rotterdam vs. Marshall; comparison of outcome predictors in traumatic brain injury using computed tomography. Revmeduas. 2021;**11**(2):87-94. DOI: 10.28960/revmeduas.2007-8013.v11.n2.002

[26] Asim M, El-Menyar A, Parchani A, Nabir S, Ahmed MN, Ahmed Z, et al. Rotterdam and Marshall scores for prediction of in-hospital mortality in patients with traumatic brain injury: An observational study. Brain Injury. 2021;**35**(7):803-811. DOI: 10.1080/02699052.2021.1927181

[27] Bm RRP, Siironen J, Skrifvars MB, Hernesniemi J, Kivisaari R. Predicting the outcome in traumatic brain injury development of a new computed tomography classification system (Helsinki CT score). Neurosurgery. 2014;**75**(6):632-647

[28] Llompart-Pou JA, Barea-Mendoza JA, Sánchez-Casado M, González-Robledo J, Mayor-García DM, et al. Neuromonitoring in severe traumatic brain injury. Data from

the Spanish ICU trauma registry (RETRAUCI). Neurosurgery. 2020;**31**(1):1-6. DOI: 10.1016/j.neucir.2019.05.005

[29] Chesnut RM, Temkin N, Carney N, et al. Global neurotrauma research group. A trial of intracranial-pressure monitoring in traumatic brain injury. The New England Journal of Medicine. 2012;**367**:2471e81. DOI: 10.1056/NEJMoa1207363

[30] Teasdale G, Maas A, Lecky F, Manley G, Stocchetti N, Murray G. The glasgow coma scale at 40 years: Standing the test of time. The Lancet Neurology. 2014;**13**(8):844-854. DOI: 10.1016/S1474-4422(14)70120-6

[31] Nyam TE, Ao KH, Hung SY, et al. Four score predicts early outcome in patients after traumatic brain injury. Neurocritical Care. 2017;**26**:225-231. DOI: 10.1007/s12028-016-0326-y

[32] Godoy DA, Rabinstein AA. How to manage traumatic brain injury without invasive monitoring? Current Opinion in Critical Care. 2022;**28**(2):111-122. DOI: 10.1097/MCC.0000000000000914

[33] Bathala L, Mehndiratta MM, Sharma VK. Transcranial doppler: Technique and common findings (part 1). Annals of Indian Academy of Neurology. 2013;**16**(2):174-179. DOI: 10.4103/0972-2327.112460

[34] Bouzat P, Oddo M, Payen J-F. Transcranial Doppler after traumatic brain injury. Current Opinion in Critical Care. 2014;**20**(2):153-160. DOI: 10.1097/mcc.0000000000000071

[35] Rasulo FA, Bertuetti R. Transcranial Doppler and optic nerve sonography. Journal of Cardiothoracic and Vascular Anesthesia. 2019;**33**:S38-S52. DOI: 10.1053/j.jvca.2019.03.040

[36] Ract C, Le Moigno S, Bruder N, Vigué B. Transcranial Doppler ultrasound goal-directed therapy for the early management of severe traumatic brain injury. Intensive Care Medicine. 2007;**33**(4):645-651. DOI: 10.1007/s00134-007-0558-6

[37] Kostin A. Transcranial Doppler in neurological intensive care. Revista Mexicana de Anestesiologia. 2015;**38**(Suppl. 3):427-429

[38] Hansen HC, Helmke K. Validation of the optic nerve sheath response to changing cerebrospinal fluid pressure: Ultrasound findings during intrathecal infusion tests. Journal of Neurosurgery. 1997;**87**:34-40. DOI: 10.3171/jns.1997.87.1.0034

[39] Ohle R, McIsaac S, Woo M, Perry J. Sonography of the optic nerve sheath diameter for detection of raised intracranial pressure compared to computed tomography. Journal of Ultrasound in Medicine. 2015;**34**(7):1285-1294. DOI: 10.7863/ultra.34.7.1285

[40] Nag DS, Sahu S, Swain A, Kant S. Intracranial pressure monitoring: Gold standard and recent innovations. World Journal of Clinical Cases. 2019;**7**(13):1535-1553. DOI: 10.12998/wjcc.v7.i13.1535

[41] Ramírez-García S, Carranza - Castro PH, Gutiérrez-Salinas J, García-Ortiz L, Hernández-Rodríguez S. Application of near-infrared spectroscopy in medicine. Medicina Interna de México. 2012;**28**(4):365-370

[42] Ghosh A, Elwell C, Smith M. Review article: Cerebral near-infrared spectroscopy in adults: A work in progress. Anesthesia and Analgesia. 2012;**115**:1373-1383. DOI: 10.1213/ANE.0b013e31826dd6a6

[43] Robba C, Santori G, Czosnyka M, Corradi F, Bragazzi N, Padayachy L, et al.

Optic nerve sheath diameter measured sonographically as non-invasive estimator of intracranial pressure: A systematic review and meta-analysis. Intensive Care Medicine. 2018;**44**(8):1284-1294. DOI: 10.1007/s00134-018-5305-7

[44] Blandino OA, Higuera JL. Usefulness of quantitative pupillometry in the intensive care unit. Medicina Intensiva. 2022;**46**(5):273-276. DOI: 10.1016/j.medine.2021.12.011

[45] Rajagopalan S, Sarwal A. Neuromonitoring in critically ill patients. Critical Care Medicine. 2023;**51**(4):525-542. DOI: 10.1097/CCM.0000000000005809

[46] Gibbs EL, Lennox W, Nims LS, Gibbs FA. Arterial and ce-rebral venous blood: Arterial-venous differences in man. The Journal of Biological Chemistry. 1942;**144**:325-332

[47] Chieregato A. Normal jugular bulb oxygen saturation. Journal of Neurology, Neurosurgery, and Psychiatry. 1 Jun 2003;**74**(6):784-786. DO: 10.1136/jnnp.74.6.784(74)49(5):583-6

[48] Aten Q, Killeffer J, Seaver C, Reier L. Causes, complications, and costs associated with external ventricular drainage catheter obstruction. World Neurosurgery. 2020;**134**:501-506. DOI: 10.1016/j.wneu.2019.10.105

[49] Nawabi NL, Stopa BM, Lassarén P, Bain PA, Mekary RA, et al. External ventricular drains and risk of freehand placement: A systematic review and meta-analysis. Clinical Neurology and Neurosurgery. 2023;**231**:107852. DOI: 10.1016/j.wneu.2019.10.105

[50] Rodríguez-Boto G, Rivero-Garvía M, Gutiérrez-González R, Márquez-Rivas J. Basic concepts about brain pathophysiology and intracranial pressure monitoring. Neurología. 2015;**30**(1):16-22. DOI: 10.1016/j.nrl.2012.09.002

[51] Teixeira PG, Inaba K, Hadjizacharia P, Brown C, Salim A, Rhee P, et al. Preventable or potentially preventable mortality at a mature trauma center. The Journal of Trauma. 2007;**63**(6):133846. DOI: 10.1097/TA.0b013e31815078ae

[52] Callcut RA, Kornblith LZ, Conroy AS, Robles AJ, Meizoso JP, Namias N, et al. The why and how our trauma patients die: A prospective Multicenter Western trauma association study. Journal of Trauma and Acute Care Surgery. 2019;**86**(5):864-870. DOI: 10.1097/TA.0000000000002205

[53] Picetti et al. WSES consensus conference guidelines: Monitoring and management of severe adult traumatic brain injury patients with polytrauma in the first 24 hours. World Journal of Emergency Surgery. 2019;**14**:53. DOI: 10.1186/s13017-019-0270-1

[54] Spahn DR, Bouillon B, Cerny V, Duranteau J, Filipescu D, Hunt BJ, et al. The European guideline on management of major bleeding and coagulopathy following trauma. Critical Care. 2017;**23**(1):98. DOI: 10.1186/s13054-019-2347-3

[55] Carney N, Totten AM, O'Reilly C, Ullman JS, Hawryluk GW, Bell MJ, et al. Guidelines for the management of severe traumatic brain injury. Neurosurgery. 2017;**80**(1):6-15. DOI: 10.1227/NEU.0000000000001432

[56] Kornblith LZ, Moore HB, Cohen MJ. Trauma-induced coagulopathy: The past, present, and future. Journal of Thrombosis and Haemostasis. 2019;**17**(6):852-862. DOI: 10.1111/jth.14450

[57] Subcommittee A. Advanced trauma life support (ATLS®). Journal of Trauma and Acute Care Surgery. 2013;**74**(5):1363-1366. DOI: 10.1097/ta.0b013e31828b82f5

[58] Badri S, Chen J, Barber J, Temkin NR, Dikmen SS, Chesnut RM, et al. Mortality and long term functional outcome associated with intracranial pressure after traumatic brain injury. Intensive Care Medicine. 2012;**38**(11):1800-1809. DOI: 10.1007/s00134-012-2655-4

[59] Bullock MR, Chesnut R, Ghajar J, Gordon D, Hartl R, Newell DW, et al. Guidelines for the surgical management of traumatic brain injury. Neurosurgery. 2006;**58**(3 Suppl.):S1-S62. DOI: 10.1227/01.NEU.0000210365.36914.E3

[60] Vik A, Nag T, Fredriksli OA, Skandsen T, Moen KG, Schirmer-Mikalsen K, et al. Relationship of "dose" of intracranial hypertension to outcome in severe traumatic brain injury. Journal of Neurosurgery. 2008;**109**(4):678-684. DOI: 10.3171/JNS/2008/109/10/0678

[61] Balestreri M, Czosnyka M, Hutchinson P, Steiner LA, Hiler M, Smielewski P, et al. Impact of intracranial pressure and cerebral perfusion pressure on severe disability and mortality after head injury. Neurocritical Care. 2006;**4**(1):8-13. DOI: 10.1385/NCC:4:1:008

[62] Bulger EM, May S, Brasel KJ, Schreiber M, Kerby JD, Tisherman SA, et al. Outof-hospital hypertonic resuscitation following severe traumatic brain injury: A randomized controlled trial. Journal of the American Medical Association. 2010;**304**(13):1455-1464. DOI: 10.1001/jama.2010.1405

[63] Geeraerts T, Velly L, Abdennour L, Asehnoune K, Audibert G, et al. Management of severe traumatic brain injury (first 24 hours). Anaesthesia, Critical Care & Pain Medicine. 2018;**37**:171-186. DOI: 10.1016/j.accpm.2017.12.001

[64] Kamel H, Navi BB, Nakagawa K, Hemphill JC 3rd, Ko NU. Hypertonic saline versus mannitol for the treatment of elevated intracranial pressure: A metaanalysis of randomized clinical trials. Critical Care Medicine. 2011;**39**(3):554-559. DOI: 10.1097/CCM.0b013e318206b9be

[65] Rickard AC, Smith JE, Newell P, Bailey A, Kehoe A, Mann C. Salt or sugar for your injured brain? A meta-analysis of randomised controlled trials of mannitol versus hypertonic sodium solutions to manage raised intracranial pressure in traumatic brain injury. Emergency Medicine Journal. 2014;**31**(8):679-683. DOI: 10.1136/emermed-2013-202679

[66] Fortune JB, Feustel PJ, Graca L, Hasselbarth J, Kuehler DH. Effect of hyperventilation, mannitol, and ventriculostomy drainage on cerebral blood flow after head injury. The Journal of Trauma. 1995;**39**(6):1091-1097. DOI: 10.1097/00005373-199512000-00014

[67] Coles JP, Minhas PS, Fryer TD, Smielewski P, Aigbirihio F, Donovan T, et al. Effect of hyperventilation on cerebral blood flow in traumatic head injury: Clinical relevance and monitoring correlates. Critical Care Medicine. 2002;**30**(9):1950-1959. DOI: 10.1097/00003246-200209000-00002

[68] Ramakrishnan V, Dahlin R, Hariri O, Quadri SA, Farr S, Miulli D, et al. Antiepileptic prophylaxis in traumatic brain injury: A retrospective analysis of patients undergoing craniotomy versus decompressive craniectomy. Surgical Neurology International. 2015;**6**:8. DOI: 10.4103/2152-7806.149613

[69] Bhullar IS, Johnson D, Paul JP, Kerwin AJ, Tepas JJ 3rd, Frykberg ER. More harm than good: Antiseizure prophylaxis after traumatic brain injury does not decrease seizure rates but may inhibit functional recovery. Journal of Trauma and Acute Care Surgery. 2014;**76**(1):54-60. DOI: 10.1097/TA.0b013e3182aafd15

[70] Roberts I, Yates D, Sandercock P, Farrell B, Wasserberg J, Lomas G, et al. Effect of intravenous corticosteroids on death within 14 days in 10,008 adults with clinically signifificant head injury (MRC CRASH trial): Randomised placebo-controlled trial. Lancet. 2004;**364**(9442):1321-1328. DOI: 10.1016/S0140-6736(04)17188-2

[71] Reinhart K, Perner A, Sprung CL, Jaeschke R, Schortgen F, Johan Groeneveld AB, et al. Consensus statement of the ESICM task force on colloid volume therapy in critically ill patients. Intensive Care Medicine. 2012;**38**(3):368-383. DOI: 10.1007/s00134-012-2472-9

[72] Stevens RD, Lazaridis C, Chalela JA. The role of mechanical ventilation in acute brain injury. Neurologic Clinics. 2008;**26**:543-563. DOI: 10.1016/j.ncl.2008.03.014

[73] Della Torre V, Badenes R, Corradi F, Racca F, Lavinio A, Matta B, et al. Acute respiratory distress syndrome in traumatic brain injury: How do we manage it? Journal of Thoracic Disease. 2017;**9**(12):5368-5381. DOI: 10.21037/jtd.2017.11.03

[74] Robba C, Camporota L, Citerio G. Acute respiratory distress syndrome complicating traumatic brain injury. Can opposite strategies converge? Intensive Care Medicine. 2023;**49**:583-586. DOI: 10.1007/s00134-023-07043-6

[75] Robba C, Poole D, McNett M, Asehnoune K, Bösel J, et al. Mechanical ventilation in patients with acute brain injury: Recommendations of the European Society of Intensive Care Medicine consensus. Intensive Care Medicine. 2020;**46**:2397-2410. DOI: 10.1007/s00134-020-06283-0

[76] Godoy DA, MurilloCabezas F, Suarez JI, Badenes R, Pelosi P, Robba C. "The Mantle" bundle for minimizing cerebral hypoxia in severe traumatic brain injury. Critical Care. 2023;**27**:13. DOI: 10.1186/s13054-022-04242-3

[77] Badjatia N. Hyperthermia and fever control in brain injury. Critical Care Medicine. 2009;**37**(Suppl):S250-S257. DOI: 10.1097/CCM.0b013e3181aa5e8d

[78] Lelubre C, Bouzat P, et al. Anemia management after acute brain injury. Critical Care. 2016;**20**:152. DOI: 10.1186/s13054-016-1321-6

[79] Taran S, Pelosi P, Robba C. Optimizing oxygen delivery to the injured brain. Current Opinion in Critical Care. 2022;**28**:145-156. DOI: 10.1097/MCC.0000000000000913

[80] Godoy DA, Lubillo S, Rabinstein AA. Pathophysiology and manage ment of intracranial hypertension and tissular brain hypoxia after severe traumatic brain injury: An integrative approach. Neurosurgery Clinics of North America. 2018;**29**:195-212. DOI: 10.1016/j.nec.2017.12.001

[81] Godoy DA, Behrouz R, Di Napoli M. Glucose control in acute brain injury: Does it matter? Current Opinion in Critical Care. 2016;**22**:120-127. DOI: 10.1097/MCC.0000000000000292

[82] Stocchetti N, Maas AI. Traumatic intracranial hypertension. The New England Journal of Medicine. 2014;**370**(22):2121-2130. DOI: 10.1056/nejmra1208708

Chapter 5

Pathways to Reduce Late Mortality of Hemorrhagic Shock

Fabrizio Giuseppe Bonanno

Abstract

Patients with progressing hemorrhagic shock (HS) die rapidly of cardiac arrest by insufficient venous return or within days by second-hit multiple organ dysfunction/failure (MOD/MOF). Once earliest source control has been effectuated and macro-hemodynamics is normalized, only three variables affect mortality, namely microcirculation, temperature, and oxygen. Late, non-immediate, mortality is usually preceded by a period of cryptic shock, essentially a disease of microcirculation in the midst of a seemingly functional macrocirculation. The persistence of the effects of ischemia-reperfusion toxemia (IRT) underlying a subclinical cryptic shock is the fundamental pathogenetic factors for clinical observed second hit deterioration. Rewarming a hypothermic hemorrhagic patient and administration of supplementary high dosages of oxygen are standard practices for the management of hemorrhagic shock in acute phase. A complete shift of paradigm prospects an answer to the above tactics' limitations, drawbacks, and contra-indications. Mild-to-moderate hypothermia, titrated supplementary oxygen, and timely-given vasodilators should instead be given during damage control surgery (DCS) for advanced shock with the aim of reducing ischemia reperfusion injury (IRI) and microcirculation dysfunction. A new strategy is suggested: preoperative hypothermia and titrated oxygen before hemorrhage source control, and intra-operative vasodilation and anti-inflammatory tactics after source control.

Keywords: hypothermia, oxygen, vasodilation, cryptic shock, acidosis, ischemia-reperfusion, MODS/MOF

1. Introduction

> *Quoting Singer and Matthay [1], "Many advances in medicine have been achieved through challenging established dogma with revolutionary thought and novel practices. Each and every specialty is reinvigorated by regular re-evaluation of processes and practices in the light of new evidence and fresh conceptualization. Challenge can galvanize fresh thinking and new approaches, yet may also reinforce and strengthen traditional paradigms if the prevailing orthodoxy is subsequently revalidated."*

1.1 Changing the paradigms

Once earliest source control has been effectuated and macro-hemodynamics is normalized, only three variables affect mortality, namely microcirculation, temperature, and oxygen.

Microcirculation optimization is crucial for prognosis of HS; hypothermia is still seen as an enemy and high flow oxygen advised in advanced HS till recently.

Can the interaction between the three variables be manipulated for improving prognosis of advanced unstable progressing HS?

2. Hypothermia in hemorrhagic shock

In hemorrhagic shock, re-warming the patient with normothermic/warm fluids and devices like the Bair Hugger is standard practice, assumedly and principally to prevent accidental hypothermia from blood loss, general anesthesia, and environmental exposure of open cavities and cold fluids [2].

Spontaneous hypothermia in hemorrhagic shock is not an independent risk factor for complications or mortality, which is correlated rather with the severity of the injury [3, 4].

Surely warming makes the patient more comfortable and prevents or stops the shivering accompanying hypothermia [5, 6], but is this practice really worthy, not to say safe [7]?

Cold increases α-adrenergic vasoconstrictive response; likewise heat increases beta-agonist response, with changes that are independent from the activity of metabolizing enzymes affected by temperature [8].

Hypothermia decreases blood flow to all organs of the body in different manner, the skeletal muscle and extremities being the most sensitive to the reduction, followed by the other internal organs, the lungs as the last. The metabolism of all drugs, in particular opioids and muscle relaxants, is slowed, and the lower is the temperature the lower and more distanced dosages are required [9].

The increase or normalization of temperature neutralizes the initial compensatory vasoconstrictive phase conveniently contributed by hypothermia, predisposing to a faster passage to a decompensated phase; moreover, hypothermia reduces the amount of fluids necessary to maintain pressure following vasoconstriction [10]. Since Hippocrates time and in World War I, it was noted that shocked patients had a higher survival when exposed to cold rather than warm environment, due to the vasoconstriction effect of cold [11].

The rationale for preventing or delaying the onset of hypothermia-related coagulopathy [12] is rather weak argument when compared to the beneficial effects on hemodynamics and metabolism in the overall computation. Hypothermia-induced coagulopathy is clinically significant at around 32°C, indicating a terminal stage of shock [5], while coagulopathy in early stage is determined by hypoxia and trauma itself, compounded by iatrogenic intervention and dilution of coagulation factors [13, 14]. Even at lower deep levels, coagulopathy remains a reversible phenomenon. In experiments on animals, spontaneous mild hypothermia does not affect coagulation in a model of controlled hemorrhagic shock [15] as predictably instead does hypothermia induced with intravenous cold solutions in uncontrolled hemorrhage models, where dilution of coagulations factors and the increased volume-driven pressures of the extra fluids become a contributing factor [16].

There is overwhelming convincing experimental evidence in animals of different size, proving the increased survival with induced intravenous and surface hypothermia compared to normothermia. This is not achieved without problems with both methods. Surface hypothermia is rather uncomfortable and intravenous fluids induce dilution coagulopathy, decreased DO_2 due to Hb curve shift to left, and must be accompanied by pharmacological control of shivering. Another drawback of surface cooling is that may accelerate death during severe hemorrhage shock because it causes reflex vasoconstriction that increases arterial pressure and bleeding speed before cooling down metabolism, which preserve cell functions [17]. For all these reasons, the systemic intravenous not-hematic fluids and surface hypothermia have been abandoned. The basic benefits of hypothermia in respect to normothermia were otherwise evident.

The experimental models of controlled hemorrhagic shock in small and big animals have confirmed the historical observations in war surgery and, ominously, the indisputable fact that hypothermia supports arterial pressure, decreases heart rate and oxygen consumption, and prevents lactate levels' rising [18–21]. It appears also to be in prospective more advantageous in advanced, uncontrolled hemorrhagic shock stages [21].

Very few studies have looked into the relation between hypothermia and hemorrhage in humans, on the claim coagulation increases bleeding by interfering with coagulation.

There is no evidence that mild hypothermia-induced coagulopathy increases mortality by increasing the rate of bleeding in elective surgery with patients kept at 36–34°C [22, 23] or in trauma patients [24], nor is evidence it increases mortality as early coagulopathy or as late coagulopathy [25, 26].

It can be postulated that the increased bleeding in the initial stages of hypothermia is consequence of vasoconstriction increasing pressure, hence bleeding rate speed, whereas in the late stages, both the vasoconstricting effect prevailing on the fading hemodynamic pump pressures and the positive effect on metabolism actually decrease mortality by preventing, slowing, or blocking further blood loss and maintaining cellular metabolism to a minimum.

A limit of the experimental studies lies in extrapolating conclusions from results obtained in laboratory on rats, dogs, and pigs, who have, respectively, much less and more fat mass than average humans, a different response to catecholamines, and a different surface-to-volume ratio. Finally, the cognitive functions tested after extracorporeal circulation are incomparable with the ones in humans [21, 27].

The main reason for the bad reputation of hypothermia in hemorrhagic shock has been the confusion between the early dynamics of spontaneous accidental hypothermia and the late metabolic hypothermia of advanced shock, between the various causes of hypothermia, and between early and late hypothermia.

Accidental, environmental, hypothermia respond to external rewarming; metabolic and cellular hypothermia does not, and only oxygenation with restoration of the capacity to produce adequate adenosine triphosphate (ATP) can reverse the latter.

2.1 Cellular effects of hypothermia

2.1.1 Protection from ischemia

ATP preservation is the essential life-preserving mechanism. ATP content is decreased in hemorrhagic shock but is regenerated once blood flow is restored in time. Cellular function remains viable up to a limit (warm ischemia period) depending on mitochondria function and up to a certain point can be re-established with restoration of perfusion [28–30].

Hypothermia diminishes the oxygen demand of the body (6–7% per 1°C cooling), protecting the most oxygen-dependent organs of the body, brain, and heart, against hypoxic damage [31]. The drop in body temperature in response to hypoxia, due to energy depletion, and a drop in heat production, unlike the ventilatory response to hypoxia, do not depend on the activation of peripheral chemoreceptors. This is the cause of metabolic hypothermia occurring in advanced HS [32].

Preservation of adenosine triphosphate (ATP) and glycogen stores in the ischemic myocardium areas, and of creatine phosphate in the non-ischemic areas appear to be as the determinant mechanisms for the benefit of hypothermia in ischemic myocardium [33, 34].

In brain cells, hypothermia reduces basal cellular metabolism by reducing oxygen uptake and consumption, with consequent shift of Hb-O_2 dissociation curve to the left and preservation of ATP content in all cells by stopping its breakdown [35, 36] and at some extent lactate and acidosis increase [37].

Ischemic neurons release neuroexcitory amines, especially glutamate, which in turn activates N-methyl-D-aspartate (NMDA) channels; once the channels are activated, calcium enters the cells and accumulates activating multiple destructive enzymes, with result of neuronal death. Hypothermia reduces the release of glutamate and another neuro-transmitter glycine needed for the NMDA receptor activation and prevents calcium entry restricting membrane permeability [38–40], so preventing cell death [41]. The reduction of calcium and lactate pathways accounts for the cell preserving effect of hypothermia in the brain.

3. Protection against ischemia-reperfusion

Hypothermia creates ischemic tolerance by several mechanisms: metabolic depression, reduced need for oxygen and energy, blundered immune and inflammatory response, and increased cell membranes tightening. Even more important is its protection from ischemia-reperfusion injury [42, 43].

Heart protection. Despite local hypothermia at 32–34°C in AMI reduces infarct size and ischemic/reperfusion damage, maintains ventricular performance and long-term remodeling, and prevents the no-reflow phenomenon, without though improving the overall outcome, its findings are ominously translatable in the prevention of IRT [44, 45].

The protective of hypothermia, whether induced or spontaneous, on I/R injury in the heart bases on the protection mitochondrial permeability transition pores, reduction of calcium overload, regulation of cellular signaling (Akt pathways, heat-shock proteins, extracellular-regulated kinase, etc.), and an overall reduction of the inflammatory response.

These events were observed when hypothermia was induced during the ischemic episode and disappeared after reperfusion [44, 45], hence the crucial importance of installing any form of therapeutic hypothermia before reperfusion.

This effect of hypothermia is timing/speed of onset-dependent. If hypothermia is present before ischemia installs can be life saving, otherwise it is not beneficial and may actually accelerate *exitus*. If tissue metabolism and heat production capacity is preserved by hypothermia before heat loss from ischemia occurs, then hypothermia is lifesaving [46–48].

Neuroprotection. The prevention and attenuation of the direct ischemic insult and the protection against ischemia-reperfusion (I-R) and ROS injury by tightening cell membranes and decreasing capillary permeability and edema in the intestinal capillaries, the most permeable in the body together with the liver and kidney ones [42, 43], are particularly useful if not crucial for brain cells IR injury or damage (IRI/D) during ROSC after successful CPR [49–53] and in neonatal encephalopathy [54–57].

Systemically induced therapeutical hypothermia (TH) at a core body temperature of 33–35°C has been shown to be beneficial not only for neonates with ischemic encephalopathy but also for comatose adults post out-of-hospital cardiac arrest with both shockable and non-shockable rhythms [54–57]. Acute brain damage from ischemia-reperfusion may further lead to other distal organ IRI [58].

Current clinical practice to prevent IRD with systemic therapeutic hypothermia involves whole-body cooling at core temperatures not below 34°C, threshold that can lead to severe complications [59–61].

Therapeutic mild hypothermia (≤34°C) reduces neurologic disability and cerebral palsy in neonatal hypoxic encephalopathy without statistically significant reductions in mortality during the neonatal period, infancy or later childhood, or in seizures at any age. Mortality at 18–24 months was though more reduced in high-income countries and not in low-income ones. The treatment should be instituted in term and late preterm infants with moderate-to-severe hypoxic ischemic encephalopathy, initiated early (within 180–360 min), and be protracted ≥48 hours [62].

Hypothermia in organ preservation. Therapeutic hypothermia (4–10°C) has been standard procedure to protect donor organs against the harmful effects of ischemia/hypoxia after surgical removal from the donor. On its own it is not enough as it increases blood viscosity, contributing to red blood cells occluding the microvasculature ("sludging") and causing detrimental microcoagulopathy. Even hemodilution did not resolve the problem [63].

This drawback stimulated the development of specialized storage solutions, integrating the hypothermic effect [64, 65].

Cellular swelling from intracellular edema at deep hypothermic levels can be explained by the temperature-dependent decrease in the activity of the Na/K-ATPase pump causing an increase in cytosolic Na + concentration and subsequent water retention. The increase of iron, ROS, and cytosol Ca++ in the first few hours of hypothermia accounts for the swelling [66, 67].

Survival in elective surgery on non-cardiovascular patients has been reported with induced temperatures down to around 5°C, around 10°C for cardiac surgery patients [68].

3.1 Clinical effects

The beneficial effects of hypothermia on heart oxygen consumption are more, the sooner the wanted temperature is reached [69].

Following the experience with deep hypothermia in thoracic aorta, a temperature target of 20°C can be seen as a safe limit for both heart and brain safety in models of extracorporeal circulation for cardiac arrest by exsanguination [70, 71]: It is safer and faster to reach than the 10°C reached with experimental big animals at a speed of 2°C/min [72].

Two-thirds of patients with trauma present with mild hypothermia, and a 10% with moderate one [73]; deep hypothermia <32°C occurs in a quarter of hypotensive shocks.

The 32°C temperature is the threshold below which significant coagulopathy occurs [5, 12, 15].

Below 26°C a rise of systemic and pulmonary vascular resistance can be noted [74].

Below 29°C dysrhythmias appear; below 24°C CA is a rule; no survival is normally the rule below 9–10°C of core temperature of spontaneous hypothermia [75].

Hypothermia decreases blood flow to all organs of the body in different manner, the skeletal muscle and extremities being the most sensitive to the reduction, followed by the other internal organs, the lungs as the last. The metabolism of all drugs, in particular opioids and muscle relaxants, is slowed so lower and more distanced doses are required, the more the lower is the temperature [9].

In ischemic hearts during mild hypothermia, the heart rate decreases while cardiac contractility is preserved, thus reducing myocardial work and oxygen consumption; the cardiac output is decreased, but the stroke volume and blood pressure are maintained.

In normal hearts, the increase in vascular resistance is caused by the increase in catecholamines release yielding to an increase of cardiac output, oxygen demand, tachycardia, and tachypnea.

With advancing hypothermia and concomitant slowing of metabolism cardiac, the cardiac output and oxygen demand decrease. Despite the protective role of hypothermia on tissue survival, profound and prolonged cooling eventually leads to circulatory failure by a direct effect on coronaries and microcirculation.

Hypothermia at 32°C in healthy coronary arteries slows coronary blood flow and increases microvascular resistance; furthermore, by increasing NO release, it exacerbates endothelium-dependent vasodilatory response. The alteration of the NO endothelium-dependent vasodilatory response makes patients with chronic ischemic heart disease and chronic heart failure prone to ischemic damage [76].

"In this pathogenetic mechanism, however, is a space for a preventive therapeutical intervention aimed to counteract coronary vasospasm and deranged excitability at core temperatures <30–29°C."

With the deepening of hypothermia, the heart slows down pumping, dysrhythmias with high risk of cardiac arrest (CA) are common with hypothermia at ≤29°C, and dysrhythmic CA with very few anecdotal exceptions is a rule <24°C. Dysrhythmias and coronary vasoconstriction is what causes CA in accidental hypothermia.

The microcirculation stagnation (no flow phenomenon) and the hemoconcentration (decreased plasma volume), due to a leakage of plasma in capillaries, cause an increase of blood viscosity and concentration and aggregation of RBC with rouleaux formation in the microcirculation, in the end contributing with the effect on the coronaries and/or myocardium to the patient's demise.

3.2 Drawbacks vs. benefits of therapeutic hypothermia

Shivering. A common drawback of hypothermia is muscle shivering: Shivering is a compensatory mechanism aimed to increase heat production. It increases oxygen demand and consumption, metabolic rate and sympathetic tone, which increase heart rate and cardiac output, and in the same time. Depleting ATP, whose hydrolysis is what produces heat. The faster the cooling is reached, however, the lesser the shivering and the oxygen consumption [77]. Shivering occurs during hypothermia induction at temperatures between 35 and 37°C and less likely at mild hypothermia between 32 and 34°C; thus, shivering may delay reaching lower target temperatures of 32–34°C and offset the therapeutic effects of hypothermia for I/R injury, pre-requisites of the therapeutical use of hypothermia [9]. Shivering disappears at temperatures <33°C [78]. Selective surface heat to hands and face, areas with the highest density of cutaneous temperature receptors, could be given *in lieu* of a pair hugger. The author recommends instead 0.3–0.5 mg/Kg of pethidine iv as safe anti-shivering drug, a sub-analgesic dose with no hypotensive effect—pethidine is already the least ventilation-depressing opioid. Morphine also settles the discomfort and has a lesser hypotensive effect and a superior sedative effect than pethidine, but has the unwanted vasodilating heat-losing effect from histamine release. Pethidine, on the other hand, has a central anti-cholinergic effect terminating rapidly the shivering that other synthetic opioids do not have; besides, rigidity and muscle spasm can show with the latter group of drugs. Interference between the drugs is a potential pitfall in terms of potentiating reciprocal side effects, *for example,* hypotension, drowsiness

Rewarming shock. Another drawback is the rewarming shock. A rewarming time > 0.25°C/h is recommended for the reheating after cardiac arrest occurring in accidental hypothermia that must be done within 6 hours. If rewarming was attempted after 5 h, experimental animals died as soon as core temperature reached 25–28°C [75]. Rewarming shock is a not well-understood complication of fast rewarming from accidental hypothermia, characterized by collapse with hypotension and tachycardia and by not progressing decrease of acidosis reverse trend. In its fulminant form, rewarming shock occurs during or shortly after rewarming and is unrelated to the occurrence of ventricular dysrhythmias. The first clinical sign is the no increase or reduction of cardiac output during rewarming, or shortly after, which is unrelated to any obvious cause, followed later by a rapid fall in blood pressure, caused by a sudden lowering of total peripheral resistance. During the process, hyperkalemia, hypoglycemia, and a rebound of increased intracranial pressure in TBI are expected.

The collapse is fatal if left untreated, but it can be buffered temporarily by interventions aimed at increasing peripheral resistance [79, 80]. It occurs only during rewarming in accidental hypothermia and does not occur during rewarming and weaning of the CPB appears.

Actual and potential benefits. If two-thirds of patients with trauma present with mild hypothermia, a 10% with moderate one [73], to bring up internal temperature up to 36°C, can be done intra-operatively fast enough in almost all patients. In experimental conditions on animals with different sizes than humans, the recommended rewarming speed from extreme temperatures of 10–15°C under CPB after induced exsanguination is 0.5°C per minute [81]. In the overall computation, hypothermia is not an enemy and has the only drawback in the shivering, causing lack of comfort in the early stages and in stopping microcirculation in advanced stages when paradoxically also a synchronous and crucially protective effect as long as the stagnation is not allowed to persist for longer than 1 maximum 6 hours [75]. Moreover, both shivering and the rewarming shock are solvable problems as is the protection of myocardium during the deepening of spontaneous accidental hypothermia when ischemia to the heart from the arrest of the pump ≤30–29°C is unwanted before deeper protective hypothermia has taken place. There is a window of therapeutical space to protect myocardium <32–30°C with rewarming and vasodilatation. The drawbacks should not hinder its beneficial applications. Hypothermia is such a relevant factor for survival at any stage of shock that no method of extreme form of resuscitation cannot disregard induced hypothermia as essential therapeutic component. Any association of causality between accidental hypothermia and mortality cannot be asserted without information on the contribution of metabolic hypothermia, *that is,* the level of macro- and micro-hemodynamics on impact, the different effects of hypothermia on macro- and microcirculation, and the timing of measurements especially in relation to the initial management of the shock and correlated hypothermia [82]. Hypothermia associated with HS is *per se* not lethal, and even its most ominous metabolic-hypoxic type, caused by hypoperfusion, could be managed with re-perfusion and intra-operative active re-warming and microcirculation vasodilatation after source control. If properly interpreted, controlled, or induced, it can only be beneficial in HS.

Timing of temperature manipulation is crucial for its benefits, as diriment is the synchronous reading of shock progression and dynamics and the distinction of the cause of hypothermia.

Moreover, systemic hypothermia with CPB is the major contributing factor to prevent or control systemic IRI [83].

The only study on the effects of hypothermia on microcirculation confirms that mild hypothermia at 34°C either protects or does not affect microcirculation. In an experiment on sheep, one group was kept in normothermia and another sent in hypothermia at 34°C with gastric circulation of cold water, both were made to bleed in a controlled volume hemorrhage. Microcirculation parameters were measured at hemodynamic stability and shock: Cortical renal, intestinal villi, and sublingual microcirculation were assessed with incident dark field illumination (IDF) video-microscopy; intestinal and renal blood flows were measured by an ultrasonic flow-meter, and mucosal PCO_2 was measured by air tonometry. Mild hypothermia does not worsen the microcirculatory derangements induced by hemorrhagic shock in the three most hit beds, with peritubular capillaries most sensitive to changes of regional and tissue perfusion than intestinal and sublingual beds [84].

4. Oxygen and hemorrhagic shock

The administration of oxygen at normobaric levels *via* a bag-mask with reservoir or an ETT with a FiO_2 of 1 (100% O_2) has been a common empiric practice in advanced shock.

It is commonly assumed that 100% oxygen, *that is,* a fraction of inspired oxygen (FiO_2) of 1 in pre-hospital setting on a patient with hypotensive hemorrhagic shock requiring intubation or the administration of 80–100% with a re-breathing mask with reservoir is good therapeutics.

There is no evidence of increased survival or of benefits with concentrations at a $FiO2 > 0.4–0.5$ in an uncontrolled hemorrhagic shock before source control, contrarily to moderate or mild hypothermia [85–87] or in controlled shock without hypoxemia [88].

As a matter of fact, hyperoxia has the opposite effect: The ischemic CNS response and the chemoreceptor response get in fact neutralized by hyperoxia in uncontrolled hemorrhage before or without source control, especially if a blood transfusion "giving a lift to that oxygen" is also running.

This might be as important reason for the better results of the "scoop and run" policy in humans and the scarce or no interference with hemodynamics before source control [89].

Oxygen in those scenarios is often given empirically without endotracheal intubation with masks with an average FiO_2 of ≤ 0.6, therefore not affecting significantly PaO_2 at the extent of neutralizing the two lifesaving reflexes.

In decompensated hypotensive shock and in absence of post-traumatic respiratory failure not requiring intercostal drain, for example, severe pulmonary contusion, patients should initially be kept at concentrations not higher than 40% FiO_2. Subsequently, 10% increases titrated to a SaO_2 of 90-94% can be effected according to arterial blood gases.

Even in a fainted patient—fainting *per se* has no correlation with HS degree, though is expected to occur often in advanced shock—PaO_2-titrated FiO_2 is required.

Total intravenous anesthesia with solely ketamine has in fact been safely done on not hemorrhagic or shocked patients and on patients with severe hemorrhages on spontaneous ventilation, breathing only oxygen-air, with no intubation or sophisticated monitoring other than clinical observations (pers. obs.).

Preoxygenation with 100% O_2 is only advised by several anesthetic societies to provide enough time during endotracheal intubation and prevent periods of hypoxia potentially occurring like difficult airway scenarios at expenses of temporary absorption atelectasis. It is also advised in CA resuscitation until ROSC.

5. Cryptic hemorrhagic shock

5.1 Ischemia-reperfusion and systemic inflammatory response

Ischemia-reperfusion phenomenon represents the continuation, local reverberation, and systemic amplification of the effects of ischemia to tissues.

Acute ischemia yields to nitrosative-oxidative stress with accumulation of by-products such as reactive oxygen and nitrogen species (ROS/RNS) that disrupts the mitochondria's enzymatic pathways and membranes, provoking an unduly intracellular accumulation of calcium, eventually leading to cell death *via* several mechanisms [90].

The stressed or dying cell itself, when reperfused, triggers an accentuation of local toxicity by calling inflammatory cells, which reverberate further damage and other cells' death. With the restoration of the circulation, toxic and inflammatory mediators are spread to remote organs [91, 92]. Preferred targets of the toxemia are the lung, the brain, the heart, the liver, and the kidney, due to their microcirculation peculiar anatomical structure.

The inflammatory mediators released as a consequence of reperfusion appear also to activate endothelial cells in remote organs that are not exposed to the initial ischemic insult. This distant response to I/R can result in leukocyte-dependent microvascular injury that is characteristic of the multiple organ dysfunction syndrome [93].

The impaired endothelium-dependent dilation in arterioles enhanced fluid filtration and leukocyte plugging in capillaries, and the trafficking of leukocytes and plasma protein extravasation in postcapillary venules.

The level of hypotension is a major determinant of the systemic inflammatory response arising during hemorrhagic shock [94]. The experimental works of Douzinas have proven the nexus between the level of ischemia and the IR-triggered inflammatory response, after previous indirect studies had correlated the level and duration of ischemia with the level of the inflammatory response [95, 96].

The phenomenon is very similar to a crush injury evolving in crush syndrome or to the toxemia and inflammatory shock following an ANP [91, 97, 98].

The gut is normally resistant to ischemia [27] but when is hit, as for its permeability, it acts as a rebound platform for a systemic spread of toxins, necrotic or inflammatory factors, and bacteria translocation even in the absence of sepsis. In a systemic IR toxemia (IRT), like the one induced by a HS, the gut is a formidable multiplier of toxemia augmented with the local bacteria translocation in addition to the inflammatory and toxic cascade. Furthermore, intestinal I/R increases luminal epithelial permeability yielding to ingress of bacteria and exit of bacteria and enterotoxins in the circulation, which can result in sepsis and multiple organ failure [99, 100].

An analogue situation occurs when the primary ischemic site is the gut itself such as in acute mesenteric ischemia or a gangrenous colon volvulus [101].

Another organ with highly permeable microcirculation, hit in any inflammatory, septic to toxic shock is the lung.

Endotoxemia in the absence of infection predisposes to infections in distant organs in the first postoperative week.

The IR local injury and systemic toxemia is not the only side effect of late inadequately treated ischemia.

A direct blunt trauma if significant or massive can give a post-traumatic inflammatory response (PTIR) of a SIR sepsis-driven, with the same endotheliopathy as underlying main pathophysiological mechanism [93, 98].

A master review describes the molecular intracellular damages induced by PTIR or post-trauma SIR after blunt trauma [102].

A reverberation and persistence of inflammatory response and endothelial dysfunction of arterioles is the underlying pathophysiological mechanism triggering a cascade of events leading to death in the first week or so.

No *restitution ad integrum* of endotheliopathy in the arterioles indicates irreversible shock [93, 98].

The resulting in increased microcirculation permeability with localized and distant organ fluid loss into the interstitial space, cytokine systemic storm and an inflammatory cascade reactions that can lead to reversible or irreversible end-organ dysfunction. Impaired endothelium-dependent dilation in arterioles, enhanced fluid and protein extravasation, platelets and leukocyte plugging in capillaries account for the clinical effects. At microcirculation capillary level, extravascular fluid hampers the transport of oxygen and decreases substrates availability, affecting all energetic processes including would dealing [102]. The reverberation between intracellular, local, regional, and systemic damage by specific intracellular and external molecules, activated in a trauma, especially a blunt one, and acting as intermediary and messengers for the SIR fuse, nonetheless the involvement *ab initio* of our innate immune system, have been postulated and prospected in a review by Pape [102].

5.2 What is cryptic shock?

The persistence of the above inflammatory, immunosuppressive, toxic, and catabolic dynamics is the reason for late, non-immediate, mortality.

Mortality after the first 6–24 hours is related to the speed and efficacy of source control, and in the first week to first month, mortality is MOD/F driven with or without sepsis [103].

The commonly used term "second hit mortality" is valid and acceptable if referred only to the timing peak of mortality. The underlying pathophysiological mechanisms are in fact a continuum [91, 98, 104, 105].

Cryptic (subclinical, persisting, silent, latent, unresolved, insidious, and refractory) hemorrhagic shock (CHS) ensues is an untreated or inadequately or late treated shock [91], carrying a 50–60% mortality [106, 107].

CHS is essentially a disease of microcirculation, where a normal macrocirculation, CaO_2, and DO_2 do not guarantee adequate VO_2 after source control or source elimination.

A situation of subclinical shock that will abut in MOD/F is then present and should be prevented, identified, and managed early before evolves *in exitus.*

Monitoring of the solely macro-hemodynamics variables may lack sufficient predictive value on the evolution of a critical patient. Often in ICU macro-hemodynamics variables are seen within normal range; nevertheless, patients still deteriorate and die all of a sudden, hit by a rapid onset multiple organ dysfunction/failure (MODS/MOF) despite reassuring values [91, 106]. It is what kills in ICU patients with normal macro-hemodynamic variables.

When macro- and microcirculation are in evident dys-synchrony [108, 109], it is essential to address the crucial role of the microcirculation/tissues interaction and hence restore physiological levels of CaO_2, DO_2, and VO_2.

Despite restoration of the macrocirculation, the sublingual microcirculation is seen impaired for at least 72 hours in hemorrhagic shock [107].

5.3 Characterization of cryptic hemorrhagic shock

Whereas in a septic or toxic shock the persisting anomaly is the persistence of sepsis factors, mediators or by-products and in a toxic shock is the underlying systemic presence of toxic and necrosis by-products [93, 98]; cryptic hemorrhagic shock is characterized by the presence of an underlying persisting ischemia-reperfusion toxemia (IRT), persisting acidosis and a dysfunctional microcirculation, and endotheliopathy in advanced stages, when the arterial gate system suffers itself of hypoxia (**Table 1**) [27, 91, 93].

Acidosis, a direct function of ischemia/hypoxia/hypoperfusion, is monitored with the rising levels, in temporal order, of NBE, LA, and pH [91, 110, 111]. Whereas ischemia-reperfusion phenomenon depends on the entity and duration of tissues relative ischemia before the index operation, acidosis is a direct function of hypoxia or infection or indicates the presence of a ischemia-reperfusion toxemia.

Different abnormalities can be observed with direct visualization of the sublingual microcirculation with hand-held vital microscopes or HVMs [orthogonal polarization spectral (OPS), sidestream dark field (SDF), and incident dark field (IDF)] in a situation of cryptic shock: spread heterogeneity of capillaries, reduced capillary density due to hemodilution and anemia, microcirculatory flow reduction due to vasoconstriction or micro-tamponade, and tissue edema [112, 113].

Other methods, such as near-infrared spectroscopy (NIRS) sublingual capnometry and cerebral oxygen saturation and skeletal muscles oxygenation, have also been used in ICU to assess microcirculation in hemorrhage, cardiac surgery, and trauma [114–120].

• Trend towards tachycardia, not explained otherwise
• MODS/MOF with normal macro-haemodynamics
• Presence of inflammatory or toxic mediators in the blood
• $\downarrow SvO_2/ScvO_2 < 65–70\%$
• NBE > 4 mmol/L
• Lactic acid >4 mmol/L
• Microcirculation imaging (spread hetereogenity of capillaries, reduced capillary density, microcirculatory flow reduction, tissue edema).

Table 1.
Characterization of cryptic shock [91].

NADPH fluorescence levels are the nearest method to measure visually tissue oxygen content [121].

> *"Clinicians never know whether optimization of the microcirculation and tissue oxygenation is actually achieved after macrovascular hemodynamic optimization. The use of automated analysis and the future possibility of introducing artificial intelligence into analysis software could eliminate observer bias and provide guidance on microvascular-targeted treatment options" [122].*

6. Prevention of second hit mortality

To prevent or limit the ischemia-reperfusion toxemia, to prevent and buffer the effects of endotheliopathy in the arteriolar system, and to adjust amount of oxygen entering the life units [98] is essential management for preventing the second hit MOD/F morbidity and mortality.

Management, therefore, must be multidirectional.

While acidosis is managed by reversing hypoxemia and rapidly controlling or eliminating the sources (stop hemorrhage in a hemorrhagic shock and remove all infected necrotic ischemic gangrenous contaminated tissues/fluids in septic shock/inflammatory shock), or optimize cardiac output (cardiogenic shock), and only at extreme levels require bicarbonate buffering, IR toxemia dynamics allow space for therapeutical strategies and manipulations in pre- and post-source control and in postoperative period.

The strategy proposed to prevent second hit IRT MODS/F can be summarized in the following: (i) the earliest or an early timed surgery preventing early mortality and the incidence and level of a second hit MOD/F; (ii) appropriate application of damage control surgery (DCS) (**Table 2**); (iii) awareness in postoperative phase of the signs characterizing the status of a cryptic subclinical shock heralding the second

Timing
Time from from injury to source control > 90-120 min in patients with haemodynamic instability
Hypotension
i Fluid-resistant hypotension or temporary (20-30 min) response to 500-1000 ml rapid infusion elicited after 2 hours from onset of a haemorrhage
ii in presence of signs of cardiac or brain ischemia
Acidosis (metabolic)/tissues hypoxia
i $ScvO_2$ < 65–70%; (ii) NBE > 6–8 mmol/L; (iii) pH < 7.2 - (values in trends).
Intra-operative reasons
i Convenience for the surgeon before transfer, ii) Unreachable bleeding, e.g. terminal ICA, high IJV, sacral vessels, retro-hepatic veins iii) Intra-Operative Hypotension, iv) Operation lasting more than 60 min on patients hemodynamically unstable before operation, v) co-presence of fecal peritonitis or of gangrenous tissues/fluids anywhere in the body, vi) tension or gap between gut and abdominal wall margins, vii) high risk of anastomosis/abdominal wall healing failure (edematous, ischemic, congested, cyanotic, not oozing margins).
THAI (timing, hypotension, acidosis, intra-operative) criteria

Table 2.
Indications for DCS [110, 111].

hit; (iv) exploiting the benefits of hypothermia preoperatively (cold blood and blood components (plasma, RBC, platelets, and no reheating)), and shivering control, (v) hypoxemic or normoxemic reperfusion post-DCS; (vi) plasma in the presence of SIR syndrome or post-traumatic inflammatory response, *for example,* in blunt trauma; (vii) reheating and vasodilatation, which has shown to be beneficial in experimental animals, intra-operatively during DCS soon after source control and pressure restoration, except if there is co-presence of severe TBI; postoperative adjuncts *pro re nata* (high doses oxygen, NO inhalation, permissive hypoxemia, cortisone/vit A, and heparin).

Once earliest source control has been effectuated and macro-hemodynamics is normalized, only three variables affect mortality, namely temperature, oxygen, and microcirculation.

6.1 Managing microcirculation

While upstream circulation derangement' correction is effected with an early or the earliest intervention of source control and venous return optimization, it is the effect of the hypoxemia distally to the tissues that determines the prognosis [123, 124].

In a progressive shock, microcirculation is put under distress and decompensates at three different moments.

First, when Crit-HbO_2 level is reached, bleeding source/s control and blood replenishment or judicious blood component restoration have not yet been accomplished.

Second, being HS, likewise CS, a vasoconstricting shock with the arteriolar reflexes system aiming to keep blood in the macrocirculation at expenses of microcirculation and tissue perfusion, when exogenous vasoconstrictors are used in the situation of a progressing hypotensive shock not responding to fluids during THR Stage III, in a phase of arterioles unresponsiveness Stage IV, or postoperatively in ICU, more distal hypoxia occurs [27, 110, 125].

Third, when circulation all of a sudden is restored and the nitrosative/oxidative stress products are enhanced and reverberated locally, and amplified systemically with damage to other organs, provided with specific special microcirculation, namely lung, liver, and kidney—the ischemia--reperfusion injury (IRI), which can become systemic ischemia-reperfusion toxemia (IRT), leading to the second hit of MODS/F.

6.2 Vasodilatation

In late phase septic shock, when vasoconstriction takes over the initial vasodilation [93], NO donors protect also against hypothermia and hypoxia/acidosis [126].

Nitroglycerin decreases systemic vascular resistance (SVR), heart work, and oxygen consumption in severe heart failure and cardiogenic shock, a vasoconstricting situation [127].

In experimental studies on small animals, low dose nitrites and other extrinsic NO donors in low doses (extrinsic acetylcholine, sodium nitroprusside, and nitroglycerin) have also shown to enhance microcirculation flow and perfusion, reverse arteriolar vasoconstriction, and increase capillary perfusion and venous return, improving central cardiac function and prevented further tissue ischemia, when administered in early, reversible, and vasoconstrictive phase of hemorrhagic shock and detrimental in late stages [128–131].

This is interpreted with the major chances of temporary timed benefits, when the arteriolar system is not in advanced hypoxemic derangement. Experimental studies were done also with animals filled with fluid after control hemorrhage and did not study a situation of pre- and post-source control. In the author's view, source control is the cut off for a rational use in humans, after restoration of pressures.

The timing of administration is therefore the key factor for a beneficial usage of vasodilators in HS.

Understanding the hemodynamics of shock (vasodilator type the septic shock in the initial phases, vasoconstrictor types the hemorrhagic, the cardiogenic and the advanced septic shock) [93] is diriment for a safe use of vasodilators.

NO donors can be administered intra-operatively, after source control and with an optimal venous return and SAP of ≥90 and MAP of ≥60 mmHg, under continuous real-time monitoring.

No hypotension should be allowed to occur intra-operatively or postoperatively.

Dosages should be titrated to maintain mean an arterial pressure (MAP) > 65–70 mm Hg under real-time continuous monitoring and a detectable response in the microcirculation. The safety of VD in SS and CS points toward a benefit in HS.

CS and HS are microcirculation vasoconstriction shocks, due to the occurring reflex response, whereas SS is vasoconstricting only un advanced stages, being a vasodilating in the initial reversible stages as for its direct effect on endothelium [93].

Intravenous infusion of vasodilators in physiological conditions has proved safe and generally beneficial in all vasoconstricting shocks, namely advanced septic shock and cardiogenic shock. In HS, intra-operative iatrogenic vasodilation soon after source control is a therefore potentially beneficial, despite a not clear mechanism.

A potential benefit of systemic infusion of nitrites or NO donors is the protective effect on patients with coronary artery disease by counteracting the vasoconstriction effect of drugs (*e.g.*, noradrenaline) and deepening hypothermia on heart and coronaries.

The benefits of a systemic vasodilatation with nitrites and NO donors have also been confirmed by NO inhalation, with its anti-inflammatory effect in preventing and counteracting the IRI to the lung, manifesting in postoperative period with secondary acute lung injury by vasoconstriction or by I-R from splanchnic organs such as gut and liver by NO [132–134].

A reduction of I-R damage in the liver from any etiology, whether primarily inflammatory or secondary hemorrhagic with NO eNOS-produced has also been noted [135].

The timing of administration with beneficial effects of iNOS inhibitors in the vasodilative phase and of NO inhalation during the vasoconstrictive phase emphasizes again the crucial importance of timing and synchronous monitoring of its effects. Areas that are lacking iNOS have less NO-induced vasodilation and become underperfused.

Vasodilation creates also an optimal micro-hemodynamics for oxygenation and removal of CO_2 buffering of acidosis and milieu normalization and IR inflammatory and toxic product removal.

Intra-operative internal and external warming under full oxygenation and after source control helps or can substitute vasodilators action. The same strategy can be applied in HS.

External warming can be added soon after source control and in postoperative period.

To bring up internal temperature up to 36°C can already be done intra-operatively. In experimental conditions on animals with different sizes than humans, the recommended warming speed from extreme temperatures of 10–15°C in large size animals is 0.5°C per minute [81].

6.2.1 Addressing ischemia-reperfusion

Systemic hypothermia and the hypoxic/ischemic post-conditioning strategy, despite the lack of clinical data pointing to a decrease in HS mortality, remain to date the best therapeutical assets available to prevent or attenuate the damage of IRI.

The benefits of hypothermia at mild moderate levels have been delineated experimentally [21].

Besides the prevention and attenuation of the direct ischemic insult, hypothermia gives protection against free radicals in I-R injury and protects against inflammation by tightening cell membranes, decreasing capillary permeability, leukotriene production, and edema [42, 43].

This effect is exploited in preventing IRI on the brain during ROSC [50, 51] in decreasing the size and performances of myocardium post-infarction [44, 45].

6.3 Systemic hypothermia pre-source control

Despite local hypothermia in AMI reduces infarct size and IRI without improving the overall outcome, its findings are ominously translatable to HS with global ischemia situation and low DO_2.

If local or regional hypothermia prevents the escalation of IR damage to heart and brain even before ischemic infarction installs, even more so systemic hypothermia may decrease the level IRD/I in HS systemic hypoperfusion and hypoxemia.

Hypothermia can be conveniently exploited preoperatively either not counteracting spontaneous accidental hypothermia or by inducing a mild-moderate level.

It should be controlled or brought and kept at the least to >30°C for drugs be effective, > 32°C to avoid the nuisance of coagulopathy requiring packing and consuming time for completion of the index operation, and below 36°C core temperature to avoid the negative effects of unnecessary high temperature in tissues that have already suffered a condition of relative hypoxia and exploit its beneficial effect on buffering IRI.

Practically, if present *ab initio*, hypothermia should not be counteracted or brought to normothermia by any means, and it should be lowered at mild-moderate levels by infusion of cold whole blood, or fresh-frozen plasma and cold RBC if the patient is normothermic.

Clinical experience with cold stored low-titer whole blood (LTWB) has been seen not to confer disadvantages on hemodynamic and safety aspects compared to normothermic blood, with the advantage of healthier platelets up to 2 weeks and higher retention of Hb at 24 hours [136–141].

If hypothermia is used as part of the treatment in HS, the entire strategy should change starting from preoperative management and anesthesia.

There is overwhelming convincing evidence in animals of different size, proving the increased survival with intravenous and surface-induced hypothermia compared with normothermia. This is not achieved without problems. Surface hypothermia would be more uncomfortable, and intravenous fluids induce dilution coagulopathy and decreased DO_2 due to Hb curve shift to left and must be accompanied by pharmacological control of shivering and in its accidental form not to be counteracted, resorting to small doses of pethidine for shivering.

Therapeutic hypothermia, after reperfusion following resuscitation with fluids, predictably cannot prolong survival in volume-controlled HS [142].

Normothermia is predictably beneficial after source control and resuscitation [143]. During surgery after source control, it is rewarming, in fact, that increases survival, and not hypothermia; likewise, it is hypothermia, which is beneficial and increases survival before source control.

In a study under volume-controlled induced HS on medium-sized animals spontaneously breathing under a GA with a vasodilating agent such as halothane, hypothermia induced after exsanguination with extracorporeal shunt cooling at 35+/−0.5°C resulted in an improved survival compared to normothermia [144]. The study was biased by the beneficial effect on the vasodilating halothane. In any case, postoperative hypothermia is not an acceptable situation or a possible iatrogenic tactics in HS. It remains beneficial in normovolemic conditions such as post-CA ROSC period or neonatal encephalopathy.

For an indirect proof of the beneficial effect of cold blood and blood components global ischemia scenario is CPB. Systemic hypothermia with CPB is the major contributing factor to prevent or control systemic IRI [49]. The different outcomes between pre- and post-source control hypothermia can be explained only by the global and more uniform distribution of hypothermia with ECLS, method not practical or convenient in postoperative period when the comfort of the patient is a main therapeutic target.

The key universal word to HS management, together with a rapid or earliest source/s control, is timing.

The protective effect of hypothermia from ischemic damage, whether induced or spontaneous, is timing/speed of onset-dependent. If hypothermia is present before ischemia installs is or maybe lifesaving, otherwise it is not beneficial and may actually accelerate *exitus*. If tissue metabolism and heat production capacity is preserved by hypothermia before heat loss from ischemia occurs, then hypothermia is lifesaving, as seen in CA from accidental hypothermia [46] and in cardioprotection post-AMI [47].

6.4 Oxygen-titrated reperfusion

Besides hypothermia, ischemia and hypoxemia have been studied to test the effects of their variations on the IR dynamics.

Excess of O_2 therapy during significant hemorrhage intensifies the physiological compensatory responses of vasoconstriction and blood flow redistribution [145]. Therefore, compared with room-air breathing, high flow or high concentration O_2 therapy deteriorates both hemodynamics and tissue/cellular hypoxia, in spite of the significantly higher arterial blood oxygenation.

Moreover, the abundance of oxygen supply in the initial phase of reperfusion produces a burst of ROS generation. This opens to the question of how possibly attenuating IRI by manipulating the oxygen content and titrate it to the cells needs.

"*Ischemic preconditioning*" is an adaptive response triggered by a brief ischemia applied before a prolonged coronary occlusion. Ischemic preconditioning (local or remote) plus antioxidants and scavengers [hypoxia-inducible factor-1α (HIF-1α) antioxidant N-acetylcysteine (NAC) antioxidant MitoQ Glutathione (GSH)] aim to prepare cells to better respond to the forthcoming stress, are difficult to apply in clinical settings, and lack effectiveness when they are applied after or during reperfusion/resuscitation [146].

The opposite tactics, "*ischemic post-conditioning*," consist in intermittent ischemia applied during early reperfusion alternating with brief periods of reperfusion [147].

A closely related technique involves initiation of transient episodes of ischemia in a remote tissue or organ at the time of reperfusion (remote *ischemic post-conditioning*). Though not advisable in HS and cardiovascular ischemia, remote "ischemic post-conditioning" confirms the advantages of ischemic/hypoxic post-conditioning in buffering, decreasing, or counteracting the side effects of IRI [148]. Resuscitation from hemorrhagic shock resulted in acute lung injury with enhanced oxidative and inflammatory pulmonary responses. However, the degree of injury correlated only with the extent of oxidative aggression [149].

A variation from the alternating cycles of ischemia-reperfusion is "*hypoxic post-conditioning*," characterized by reperfusion under normoxia alternated with periods of hypoxia. The tactic was found to reduce the formation of reactive oxygen species (ROS), lipid membrane peroxidation, and intracellular and mitochondrial Ca(2+) overload [150].

"*Hypoxemic resuscitation*" with PaO_2 at 35–40 mmHg compared to normoxemic resuscitation with PaO_2 at 95–105 mmHg has been seen attenuating lactate production, lower ROS production, lesser oxidative and inflammatory stress [151], and pulmonary capillary endothelial dysfunction in respect of normoxemia in medium-size animals such as rabbits, following induced volume-controlled HS [152].

Hypoxemic reperfusion consists in gradually increasing initially during reperfusion the FiO_2 of the reperfusate from a lower level at PaO_2 levels of 30–35 mmHg to PaO_2 levels of 95–105 mmHg at the end of the resuscitation period. At a PaO_2 range between 35 and 130 mm Hg no significant metabolite concentration changes are seen [153]. Though tested only in experimental settings, the new conceptual development, revamped from a combination of the experimented "hypoxic post-conditioning and hypoxemic resuscitation" tactics, represents the most conceptually optimal method for oxygenating tissues without increasing the IRI [154].

The advantage of ischemic position is in the possibility to modulate PaO_2 using different levels of FiO_2 without compromising perfusion. In this way, ROS and the intracellular pH are kept at a minimum, at the same time oxygen is available to mitochondria for ATP generation/storing, and metabolic waste is not slowed.

Another potential advantage of hypoxemic reperfusion compared to the use of antioxidants is that it aims to prevent ROS production rather than eliminate their deleterious effects.

Moreover, hypoxemic reperfusion may be advantageous compared to post-conditioning strategies since blood flow is restored offering better replenishment from metabolic wastes.

Two experimental studies highlight the relevance of oxygenation on the perfusion in determining IRI and overall prognosis in resuscitation of a progressive hemorrhagic shock.

In a study, tissue oxygenation (PO_2 e tPO_2) improved at a FiO_2 of 1 in normovolaemia and at blood volume losses of less than 20%. Instead, at significant, for more than 50% blood volume losses, high inspired oxygen admixtures lead to precipitous reduction of tissue oxygenation, similar to that of animals breathing in-room air. An even worse outcome was observed by inducing hypoxemia (breathing at FiO_2 = 0.15) without resuscitation; all parameters deteriorated, and the animals had an earlier death. Hypoxemia combined with hypoperfusion accelerated the tPO_2 fall considerably [155].

An experiment *in vitro* on cardiomyocytes from explanted heart has shown that exposure to hypoxemic and room oxygen levels over a 72-h period results in significantly lower amounts of pro-inflammatory cytokine release than intermittent or continuous hyperoxia. Cardiac myocytes obtained from the explanted hearts were exposed to constant hyperoxia (95% O_2), intermittent hyperoxia (alternating 10-min exposures to 5 and 95% O_2), constant normoxia (21% O_2), or constant mild hypoxia (5% O_2), using a bioreactor. Constant and intermittent hyperoxia induced inflammation and cytotoxicity soon after exposure, which was the greatest after constant hyperoxia and even brief hyperoxic episodes [156].

In the last 7 years there has not been any study or *in vivo* application of hypoxemic reperfusion tailoring oxygen administration to HS level.

Only one study has showed that the more advanced is shock, the lesser oxygen is required. In it, where rats were made to bleed 70% of their TBV in a controlled HS experiment, a 3-week-old hypoxically stored RBCs, made hypoxic using an O_2 depletion system, scored like fresh RBC and better than conventional 3-week-old stored RBC in terms of hemodynamics and organ injury, during resuscitation, and in terms of oxidative stress, RNA/DNA injury, and lipid per oxidation, following reperfusion [157].

6.5 Normothermic plasma

Trauma causes a systemic inflammatory response, which, contrarily to sepsis and inflammatory shock [91, 98] where is regularly and primarily hit, in trauma with or without hemorrhage is more present in severe blunt trauma, due to the relative increased response for the relative increase of soft tissue injuries in respect to a penetrating one where the inflammatory reaction is present only mainly along the track of the offense weapons trajectories. Moreover, SIR messengers and factors are lost in a relative bigger amount in a penetrating trauma than a blunt one where tissue contusions are universally present compared to a penetrating trauma. Endothelial cell damage and glycocalyx shedding of capillaries and arterioles are the main target, yielding to coagulopathy, further inflammation, increased vascular permeability, and dyslexia that may lead to death. The microcirculation derangement is mirrored by worsening of flow, density, and heterogeneity of capillaries within microvessels, as seen with sublingual incident dark field video-microscopy [158].

The vascular endothelium plays a central role in maintaining organ homeostasis through its regulation of vascular tone, coagulation, inflammation, and barrier function and the vital interaction with the distal tissues on gas exchange. Dysregulation of normal endothelial function occurs during major injuries with severe tissues trauma, hemorrhagic shock, and burns, where it gives rise to systemic microvascular thrombosis, inflammation, loss of barrier integrity, coagulopathy, and respiration dysregulation. The endotheliopathy of trauma involves a complex interplay between the glycocalyx, von Willebrand factor (VWF), expressed on its surface, and platelets. Upon exposure to subendothelial proteins such as collagen, VWF binds platelets to the injured vasculature. The endothelium, which provides an anticoagulant and platelet-repellent surface in the resting state, becomes highly procoagulant and attracts platelets and leukocytes when its protective glycocalyx is depleted. Hyperadhesive VWF also binds leukocytes to normal ECs remote from the injury site [159].

Normothermic FFP is the most effective fluid in restoring the endothelial glycocalyx and junctions, in reducing endothelial permeability, and in attenuating the early inflammation/coagulation response. The mechanism is not clear but is likely due to the effects of the several components of FFP as the same beneficial effects have been seen also with plasma-derived products such as prothrombin complex concentrate (PCC) and lyophilized and spray-dried plasma. The protective effects of FFP are diminished by post-thaw storage at 4°C for 5 days and are time sensitive with most efficacy with the first 3 hours post trauma [160].

A decrease of 30 days mortality was found with plasma when compared to no plasma, but only in blunt trauma [161]. In some blunt trauma, such as a predominantly orthopedic blunt poly-trauma a variable post-traumatic inflammatory response ensues. In these scenarios, the inflammatory cascade has more chance of being retained inside circulation, damaging the endothelium and microcirculation, than a penetrating trauma where the inflammatory avalanche gets lost with the blood loss. Presumably, following the loss of inflammatory or toxic mediators and factors with the blood loss, there is a notable absence or a comparably lesser amount of SIR and IRT in penetrating injury, while the post-traumatic inflame response is very much present and longer lasting in a blunt injury where viable but damaged tissue contusions or hematoma continue being a source of SIR or IRT. This explains why plasma has benefits in blunt injury when added to blood.

Another advantage of plasma in blunt trauma is that it helps the release of VWF from ECs. This action is prevented by the anti-fibrinolytic agent tranexamic acid, providing a direct link between endotheliopathy and fibrinolysis during acute trauma [162].

These findings make normothermic plasma an important fluid in postoperative management of a HS from a blunt poly-trauma. An advantage can further come in decreasing plasma amenable coagulopathies, if already present and missed.

6.6 Postoperative therapeutic adjuncts

Cortisone is the perfect drug for curbing lung inflammation in the initial stages of secondary ALI by any etiology as well as any inflammatory microcirculation derangement of kidney and liver.

Cortisone has two major potentially negative side effects in the immediate postoperative period: healing interference and impairment, and curbing the inflammatory response to IRI/T. While healing is not impaired if given in the first 3 days, not anyway enough to interfere with healing processes of an anastomosis or abdominal/chest wall union, and can anyhow be counteracted by high doses of vitamin A, its anti-inflammatory property is a major problem. Its use with intent to prevent or curb the IRI to lungs kidneys and liver needs to be well pondered.

Heparin until mobilization remains another option practicable with a predictive and preventive therapeutical role in early IRI. Heparin small doses could be added to dissolve microthrombi in microcirculation especially in the lung we have seen to be an important pathogenetic mechanism for the VQ mismatch of interstitial pneumonia or ALI/ARDS occurring in second hit MOD/F. This effect must be plot against wound mucosal anastomosis oozing in patients with mild or moderate TBI [25, 26].

Therapeutic oxygen at concentrations above FiO_2 of 0.6 in a HS has to be considered as normobaric hyperoxia and avoided, in both preoperative and postoperative periods. It has been seen that 40–50% equals 100% in terms of oxygenation without the side effects of hypoxemia; 60% is therefore the maximum that should be given in a HS for oxygenation purposes. Higher concentrations should be considered only for special purposes, *for example,* CA initial resuscitation until ROSC or concomitant acute respiratory failure by added pulmonary trauma. Despite a proven anti-inflammatory and anti-infection property in experimental settings [163], it is not clear as to which patients and or which conditions would benefit of hypoxemia to decrease postoperative surgical site infections' rates [164]. Certainly, oxygen is necessary for healing and prevention of infection: Oxidative bursts of neutrophils require molecular O_2 [165, 166]. Oxygen in high doses PaO_2 > 60% can be necessary, if the tiO_2 and VO_2 could be reliably calculated prn. VO_2, in fact, is not an accurate index of tissutal PaO_2 under conditions of tissue hypoxia [167]. A possible benefit on post-operative infections' prevention cannot be excluded either.

The damages to lung alveoli microcirculation and structure due to vasoconstriction and the excess of ROS at superior normobaric doses are the drawback to avoid.

Hyperbaric oxygen is not an option too.

Inhaled NO can be used in ICU for preventing secondary ALI or the lung microcirculation vasoconstriction [131–134].

6.7 Permissive hypoxemia

Mild permissive hypoxemia (PaO_2 55–80 mmHg; SpO_2 88–92%) results in improved outcomes also in patients at risk or with actual early acute lung injury, included those with ARDS or with ARF from other causes. Preliminary results with low FiO_2 at 0.5 in a mix population have confirmed the safety and therapeutic efficacy of a "permissive hypoxemia" tactics, with improvement of in-hospital mortality, a longer ventilator-free day period, and an improvement of the 28-day mortality in an ARDS subset and a worse outcome in high or hypoxemic concentrations [168].

7. Perspective

On these bases, a strategy can be drawn for timely application before or soon after source control in an advanced shock requiring DCS [111], when IR toxemia and cryptic shock are very likely to install and determine prognosis (**Table 3**).

The framework conceptualized by Convertino of a similarity between extreme physical exercise requiring increasing VO_2 and the need to ensure sufficient VO_2 after normalization of CaO_2 and DO_2 [169] as well as the conclusions of a study by Gutierrez et al. showing clearly high FiO_2 cannot compensate for the low cardiac output and absence of tissue perfusion and O_2 transport does not necessarily correlate with sufficient or optimal VO_2 that is in fact limited only by the diffusion of oxygen from capillaries to cells [167] and address the crucial questions and research directions to follow, if we want to diminish late HS mortality by preventing, buffering, and managing the pathophysiological mechanisms leading to *exitus*.

The real-time *in vivo* monitoring of microcirculation [122] remains essential in the first three-hour days postop, when full-blown cryptic shock installs develop and can be timely managed.

BEFORE SOURCE CONTROL Preop./Intraop.	AFTER SOURCE CONTROL Intraop.	POST-OPERATIVE ICU Options
Leave Oxygen at room air with a calculated blood loss of 40% TBV or in presence of heart or brain sign of ischemia.	Use vasodilators under intra-operative monitoring after source control and pressures restoration.	Cortisone
Give Oxygen with an initial FiO_2 of 0.4 with 10% increases titrated to a SaO_2 of 90-94% if shock not responding to fluid-load test – Stage III & IV Physiological Classification of HS.	Use hypoxaemic post-conditioning reperfusion with alternate cycles of normoxia at 35-40 mm Hg and 100 mm Hg of PaO_2 x 72-96 hours.	Heparin
No rewarming but leave at spontaneous hypothermia level or induced hypothermia at mild-moderate level (>33<36°).	Rewarm the patient intra-operatively soon after source control and pressures restoration.	Therapeutic Oxygen
Cold blood or blood components	Use normothermic plasma in blunt trauma or if concomitant presence of contaminated or infected or necrotic or gangrenous tissues/fluids was also done.	Inhaled Nitric Oxide
		Permissive Hypoxaemia

Table 3.
Strategies.

Author details

Fabrizio Giuseppe Bonanno
Department of Surgery, Polokwane Provincial Hospital, Polokwane, South Africa

*Address all correspondence to: f.g.bonanno@gmail.com

References

[1] Singer M, Matthay MA. Clinical review: Thinking outside the box – An iconoclastic view of current practice. Critical Care. 2011;**15**:225

[2] Rauch S, Miller C, Bräuer A, Wallner B, Bock M, Paal P. Perioperative hypothermia-a narrative review. International Journal of Environmental Research and Public Health. 2021;**18**:8749

[3] Mommsen P, Andruszkow H, Frömke C, Zeckey C, Wagner U, van Griensven M, et al. Effects of accidental hypothermia on posttraumatic complications and outcome in multiple trauma patients. Injury. 2013;**44**:86-90

[4] Nishi K, Takasu A, Shinozaki D, Sakamoto K, Yamamoto Y, Sakamoto T. Hypothermia does not hasten death during uncontrolled hemorrhagic shock presenting as the "triad of death" in rats. Acute Medicine & Surgery. 2015;**2**:29-34

[5] Jurkovich GJ, Greiser WB, Luterman A, Curreri PW. Hypothermia in trauma victims: An ominous predictor of survival. The Journal of Trauma. 1987;**27**:1019-1024

[6] Gentilello LM, Jurcovich GJ, Stark MS, Hassantash SA, O'Keefe GE. Is hypothermia in the victim of major trauma protective or harmful? Annals of Surgery. 1997;**226**:439-447

[7] Convertino VA, Cap AP. Should patients with haemorrhage be kept warm? The Journal of Physiology. 2010;**588**(Pt. 17):3135

[8] Matheny JL, Ahlquist RP. Role of neuronal and extraneuronal factors in temperature mediated responsiveness of adrenoceptors. Archives Internationales de Pharmacodynamie et de Thérapie. 1976;**224**:180-189

[9] Jung KT, Bapat A, Kim Y-K, Hucker WJ, Lee K. Therapeutic hypothermia for acute myocardial infarction: A narrative review of evidence from animal and clinical studies. Korean Journal of Anesthesiology. 2022;**75**:216-230

[10] Nishi K, Takasu A, Shibata M, Uchino S, Yamamoto Y, Sakamoto T. Hypothermia reduces resuscitation fluid volumes required to maintain blood pressure in a rat Hemorrhagic shock model. The Journal of Trauma. 2012;**72**:130-135

[11] Swan H. Clinical hypothermia: A lady with a past and some promise for the future. Surgery. 1973;**73**:736-758

[12] Gubler KD, Gentilello LM, Hassantash SA, Maier RV. The impact of hypothermia on diluitional coagulopathy. The Journal of Trauma. 1994;**36**:847-851

[13] Brohi K, Cohen MJ, Ganter MT, Schultz MJ, Levi M, Mackersie RC, et al. Acute coagulopathy of trauma: hypoperfusion induces systemic anticoagulation and hyperfibrinolysis. The Journal of Trauma. 2008;**64**:1211-1217

[14] Floccard B, Rugeri L, Faure A, Denis MS, Boyle EM, Peguet O, et al. Early coagulopathy in trauma patients: An on-scene and hospital admission study. Injury. 2010;**43**:26-32

[15] Iwamoto S, Takasu A, Sakamoto T. Therapeutic mild hypothermia: Effects on coagulopathy and survival in a rat hemorrhagic shock model. The Journal of Trauma. 2010;**68**:669-675

[16] Wu X, Kochanek PM, Cochran K, Nozari A, Henchir J, Stezoski SW, et al. Mild hypothermia improves survival after prolonged, traumatic hemorrhagic shock in pigs. The Journal of Trauma. 2005;**59**:291-301

[17] Takasu A, Ishihara S, Anada H, Sakamoto T, Okada Y. Surface cooling, which fails to reduce the core temperature rapidly, hastens death during severe hemorrhagic shock in pigs. The Journal of Trauma. 2000;**48**:942-947

[18] Takasu A, Norio H, Sakamoto T, Okada Y. Mild hypothermia prolongs the survival time during uncontrolled hemorrhagic shock in rats. Resuscitation. 2002;**54**:303-309

[19] Wu X, Stezoski J, Safar P, Nozari A, Tisherman SA. After spontaneous hypothermia during hemorrhagic shock, continuing mild hypothermia (34 degrees C) improves early but not late survival in rats. The Journal of Trauma. 2003;**55**:308-316

[20] George ME, Mulier KE, Bellman GJ. Hypothermia is associated with improved outcomes in a porcine model of hemorrhagic shock. The Journal of Trauma. 2010;**68**:662-668

[21] Hildebrand F, Radermacher P, Ruchholtz S, Huber-Lang M, Seekamp A, Flohè S, et al. Relevance of induced and accidental hypothermia after trauma-haemorrhage. Intensive Care Medicine Experimental. 2014;**2**:16

[22] Schmied H, Kurz A, Sessler DI, Kozek S, Reiter A. Mild hypothermia increases blood loss and transfusion requirements during total hip arthroplasty. Lancet. 1996;**3**:289-292

[23] Rajagopalan S, Mascha E, Na J, Sessler DI. The effects of mild perioperative hypothermia on blood loss and transfusion requirement. Anesthesiology. 2008;**108**:71-77

[24] Lester ELW, Fox E, Holcomb JB, Brasel K, Bulger E, Cohen MJ, et al. The impact of hypothermia on outcomes in massively transfused patients. Journal of Trauma and Acute Care Surgery. 2019;**86**:458-463

[25] Bonanno FG. Early coagulopathy in trauma and major bleeding: Is it time to challenge the dogma? Trauma. 2021;**1**:1-4

[26] Bonanno F. Facts and myths of coagulopathies in trauma and major bleeding - to clear the fog. In: Advancement and New Understanding in Medical Sciences. Vol. 3. Ch 6. Bengal, India. 2023. DOI: 10.9734/bpi/anums/v3/7338C

[27] Bonanno FG. Hemorrhagic shock: The physiology approach. Journal of Emergencies, Trauma, and Shock. 2012;**5**:285-295

[28] Marubayashi S, Takenaka M, Dohi K, Ezaki H, Kawasaki T. Adenine nucleotide metabolism during hepatic ischemia and subsequent blood reflow periods and its relation to organ viability. Transplantation. 1980;**30**:294-296

[29] Chaudry IH. Cellular mechanisms in shock and ischemia and their correction. The American Journal of Physiology. 1983;**14**:R117-R134

[30] Storey KB, Storey JM. Tribute to P. L. Lutz: Putting life on 'pause' – Molecular regulation of hypometabolism. The Journal of Experimental Biology. 2007;**210**:1700-1714

[31] Wood S. Interactions between hypoxia and hypothermia. Annual Review of Physiology. 1991;**53**:71-85

[32] Steiner AA, Branco LGS. Hypoxia-induced anapyrexia: Implications and

putative mediators. Annual Review of Physiology. 2002;**64**:263-288. DOI: 10.1146/annurev.physiol.64.081501.155856

[33] Hale SL, Kloner RA. Myocardial temperature in acute myocardial infarction: Protection with mild regional hypothermia. The American Journal of Physiology. 1997;**273**:H220-H227

[34] Simkhovich BZ, Hale S, Kloner RA. Metabolic mechanism by which mild regional hypothermia preserves ischemic tissue. Journal of Cardiovascular Pharmacology and Therapeutics. 2004;**9**:83-90

[35] Stone GH, Donnelly C, Frobese AS. The effect of lowered body temperature on the cerebral hemodynamics and metabolism of man. Surgery, Gynecology & Obstetrics. 1956;**103**:313-317

[36] Kramer AS, Sanders AP, Lesage AM, Woodhall B, Sealy WC. The effect of profound hypothermia on preservation of cerebral ATP content during circulatory arrest. The Journal of Thoracic and Cardiovascular. 1968;**56**:699-709

[37] Erecinska M, Thoresen M, Silver IA. Effects of hypothermia on energy metabolism in mammalian central nervous system. Journal of Cerebral Blood Flow and Metabolism. 2003;**23**:513-530

[38] Rothman SM, Olney JW. Glutamate and the pathophysiology of hypoxic-ischemic brain damage. Annals of Neurology. 1986;**19**:105-111

[39] Busto R, Globus MY-T, Dietrich WD, Martinez E, Valdes I, Ginsberg MD. Effect of mild hypothermia on ischemia-induced release of neurotransmitters and free fatty acids in rat brain. Stroke. 1989;**20**:904-910

[40] Gonzalez-Ibarra FP, Varon J, Lopez-Meza EG. Therapeutic hypothermia: A critical review the molecular mechanisms of action. Frontiers in Neurology. 2011;**2**:4

[41] Ding D, Moskowitz SI, Li R, Lee SB, Esteban M, Tomaselli K, et al. Acidosis induces necrosis and apoptosis of cultured hippocampal neurons. Experimental Neurology. 2000;**162**:1-12

[42] Jurkovich GJ, Pitt RM, Curreri PW, Granger DN. Hypothermia prevents increased capillary permeability following ischemia-reperfusion injury. The Journal of Surgical Research. 1988;**44**:514-521

[43] Childs EW, Udobi KF, Hunter FA. Hypothermia reduces microvascular permeability and reactive oxygen species expression after hemorrhagic shock. The Journal of Trauma. 2005;**58**:2

[44] Kohlhauer M, Berdeaux A, Ghaleh B, Tissier R. Therapeutic hypothermia to protect the heart against acute myocardial infarction. Archives of Cardiovascular Diseases. 2016;**109**:716-722

[45] Yamada KP, Kariya T, Aikawa T, Ishikawa K. Effects of therapeutic hypothermia on Normal and ischemic heart. Frontiers in Cardiovascular Medicine. Feb 2021;**15**(8):642843. DOI: 10.3389/fcvm.2021.642843

[46] Gilbert M, Busund R, Skagseth A, Nilsen PA, Solbø JP. Resuscitation from accidental hypothermia of 13.7 degrees C with circulatory arrest. Lancet. 2000;**355**(9201):375-376

[47] Kanemoto S, Matsubara M, Noma M, Leshnower BG, Parish LM, Jackson BM, et al. Mild hypothermia to limit myocardial ischemia-reperfusion injury: Importance of timing. The Annals of Thoracic Surgery. 2009;**87**:157-163

[48] Erlinge D, Götberg M, Noc M, Lang I, Holzer M, Clemmensen P, et al. Therapeutic hypothermia for the treatment of acute myocardial infarction-combined analysis of the RAPID MI-ICE and the CHILL-MI trials. Therapeutic Hypothermia and Temperature Management. 2015;**5**:77-84

[49] Tahsili-Fahadan P, Farrokh S, Geocadin RG. Hypothermia and brain inflammation after cardiac arrest. Brain Circulation. Jan-March 2018;**4**(1):1-13. Available from: http://www.braincirculation.org. DOI: 10.4103/bc.bc_4_18

[50] Sandroni C, Cronberg T, Sekhon M. Brain injury after cardiac arrest: Pathophysiology, treatment, and prognosis. Intensive Care Medicine. 2021;**47**(12):1393-1414

[51] Doherty DR, Parshuram CS, Gaboury I, Hoskote A, Lacroix J, Tucci M, et al. Hypothermia therapy after pediatric cardiac arrest. Circulation. 2009;**119**:1492-1500

[52] He S, Weng Y, Sun S, Chen W, Wu X, Li Z, et al. Comparison of the durations of mild therapeutic hypothermia on outcome after cardiopulmonary resuscitation in the rat. Circulation. 2012;**125**:123-129

[53] Lindsay PJ, Buell D, Scales DC. The efficacy and safety of pre-hospital cooling after out-of-hospital cardiac arrest: A systematic review and meta-analysis. Critical Care. 2018;**22**:66

[54] Cotten CM, Shankaran S. Hypothermia for hypoxic-ischemic encephalopathy. Expert Review of Obstetrics and Gynecology. 2010;**5**:227-239

[55] Ma H, Sinha B, Pandya RS, Lin N, Popp AJ, Li J, et al. Therapeutic hypothermia as a neuroprotective strategy in neonatal hypoxic-ischemic brain injury and traumatic brain injury. Current Molecular Medicine. 2012;**12**:1282-1296

[56] Chang M. Therapeutic hypothermia for newborns with hypoxic ischemic encephalopathy. Neonatal Medicine. 2013;**20**:2-11

[57] Zhang XW, Xie JF, Chen JX, Huang YZ, Guo FM, Yang Y, et al. The effect of mild induced hypothermia on outcomes of patients after cardiac arrest: A systematic review and meta-analysis of randomised controlled trials. Critical Care. 2015;**19**:417

[58] Robba C, Battaglini D, Samary CS, Silva PL, Ball L, Rocco PRM, et al. Ischaemic stroke-induced distal organ damage: Pathophysiology and new therapeutic strategies. Intensive Care Medicine Experimental. 2020;**8**:23

[59] Polderman KH. Mechanisms of action, physiological effects, and complications of hypothermia. Critical Care Medicine. 2009;**37**:S186-S202

[60] Vaity C, Al-Subaie N, Cecconi M. Cooling techniques for targeted temperature management post-cardiac arrest. Critical Care. 2015;**19**:103

[61] Nolan JP, Sandroni C, Bottiger BW, Cariou A, Cronberg T, Friberg H, et al. European resuscitation council and European society of intensive care medicine guidelines 2021: Post-resuscitation care. Resuscitation. 2021;**161**:220-269

[62] Mathew JL, Kaur N, Dsouza JM. Therapeutic hypothermia in neonatal hypoxic encephalopathy: A systematic review and meta-analysis. Journal of Global Health. 2022;**12**:04030

[63] Taylor MJ, Bailes JE, Elrifai AM, Shih SR, Teeple E, Leavitt ML, et al.

A new solution for life without blood. Asanguineous low-flow perfusion of a whole-body perfusate during 3 hours of cardiac arrest and profound hypothermia. Circulation. 1995;**91**:431-444

[64] Roskott AMC, Nieuwenhuijs VB, Dijkstra G, Koudstaal LG, Leuvenink HGD, Ploeg RJ. Small bowel preservation for intestinal transplantation: A review. Transplant International. 2011;**24**:107-131

[65] Michel SG, Madsen JC. Current perspectives in transplant medicine: Hypothermic oxygenated perfusion. Transplant Research and Risk Management. 2016;**8**:25-30

[66] Petrat F, de Groot H, Sustmann R, Rauen U. The chelatable iron pool in living cells: A methodically defined quantity. Biological Chemistry. 2002;**383**:489-502

[67] Rauen U, de Groot H. Mammalian cell injury induced by hypothermia - the emerging role for reactive oxygen species. Biological Chemistry. 2002;**383**:477-488

[68] Stephen CR, Dent SJ, Hall KD, Smith WW. Physiologic reactions during profound hypothermia with cardioplegia. Anesthesiology. 1961;**22**:873-881

[69] Ziganshin BA, Elefteriades JA. Deep hypothermic circulatory arrest. Annals of Cardiothoracic Surgery. 2013;**2**:303-315

[70] Mohiyaddin S, Nanjaiah P, Saad AO, Acharya MN, Khan TA, Davies RH, et al. Suspended animation: The past, present and future of major cardiothoracic trauma. ANZ Journal of Surgery. 2018;**88**:678-682

[71] Moffatt SE, Mitchell SJB, Walke JL. Deep and profound hypothermia in haemorrhagic shock, friend or foe? A systematic review. Journal of the Royal Army Medical Corps. 2018;**164**:191-196

[72] Alam HB, Chen Z, Honma K, Koustova E, Querol RI, Jaskille A, et al. The rate of induction of hypothermic arrest determines the outcome in a swine model of lethal hemorrhage. The Journal of Trauma. 2004;**57**:961-969

[73] Tsuei BJ, Kearney PA. Hypothermia in the trauma patient. Injury. 2004;**35**:7-15

[74] Cooper KE, Hunter AR, Keatinge WR. Accidental hypothermia. International Anesthesiology Clinics. 1964;**24**(2):999-1014

[75] Lott C, Truhla A, Alfonzo A, Barelli A, Gonzalez-Salvado V, Hinkelbein J, et al. European resuscitation council guidelines 2021: Cardiac arrest in special circumstances. Resuscitation. 2021;**161**:152-219

[76] Bobi J, Solanes N, Dantas AP, Ishida K, Regueiro A, Castillo N, et al. Moderate hypothermia modifies coronary Hemodynamics and endothelium-dependent vasodilation in a porcine model of temperature management. Journal of the American Heart Association. 2020;**9**(3):e014035. DOI: 10.1161/JAHA.119.014035

[77] Taniguchi Y, Lenhardt R, Sessler DI, Kurz A. The effect of altering skin-surface cooling speeds on vasoconstriction and shivering thresholds. Anesthesia and Analgesia. 2011;**113**:540-544

[78] Polderman KH, Herold I. Therapeutic hypothermia and controlled normothermia in the intensive care unit: Practical considerations, side effects, and cooling methods. Critical Care Medicine. 2009;**37**:1101-1120

[79] Tveita T, Ytrehus K, Myhre ESP, Hevrøy O. Left ventricular dysfunction following rewarming from experimental hypothermia. Journal of Applied Physiology. 1998;**85**(6):2135-2139

[80] Scaravilli V, Bonacina D, Citerio G. Rewarming: Facts and myths from the systemic perspective. Critical Care. 2012;**16**:A25

[81] Alam HB, Rhee P, Honma K, Chen H, Ayuste EC, Lin T, et al. Does the rate of rewarming from profound hypothermic arrest influence the outcome in a swine model of lethal hemorrhage? The Journal of Trauma. 2006;**60**:134-146

[82] Rösli D, Schnüriger B, Candinas D, Haltmeier T. The impact of accidental hypothermia on mortality in trauma patients overall and patients with traumatic brain injury specifically: A systematic review and meta-analysis. World Journal of Surgery. 2020;**44**(12):4106-4117

[83] Rosenthal LM, Tong G, Wowro S, Walker C, Pfitzer C, Böttcher W, et al. A prospective clinical trial measuring the effects of cardiopulmonary bypass under mild hypothermia on the inflammatory response and regulation of cold-shock protein RNA-binding motif 3. Therapeutic Hypothermia and Temperature Management. 2020;**10**(1):60-70

[84] Caminos Eguillor JF, Ferrara G, Kanoore Edul VS, Buscetti MG, Canales HS, Lattanzio B, et al. Microcirculatory effects of rewarming in experimental hemorrhagic shock. Microvascular Research 2023;**147**:104490. Epub 2023 January 31. DOI: 10.1016/j.mvr.2023.104490

[85] Kim SH, Stezoski SW, Safar P, Fisherman SA. Hypothermia, but not 100% oxygen breathing, prolongs survival time during lethal uncontrolled hemorrhagic shock in rats. The Journal of Trauma. 1998;**44**:485-491

[86] Takasu A, Stezoski SW, Stezoski J, Safar P, Tisherman SA. Mild or moderate hypothermia, but not increased oxygen breathing, increases long-term survival after uncontrolled hemorrhagic shock in rats. Critical Care Medicine. 2000a;**28**:2465-2474

[87] Takasu A, Iwamoto S, Ando S, Minagawa Y, Kashiba M, Yamamoto Y, et al. Effects of various concentrations of inhaled oxygen on tissue disoxia, oxidative stress, and survival in a rat hemorrhagic shock model. Resuscitation. 2009;**80**:826-831

[88] Takasu A, Prueckner S, Tisherman SA, Stezoski SW, Stezoski J, Safar P. Effects of increased oxygen breathing in a volume controlled hemorrhagic shock outcome model in rats. Resuscitation. 2000;**45**:209-220

[89] Bickell WH, Wall MJ, Pepe PE, Martin RR, Ginger VF, Allen MK, et al. Immediate versus delayed fluid resuscitation for hypotensive patients with penetrating torso injuries. The New England Journal of Medicine. 1994;**331**:1105-1109

[90] Carden DL, Granger DN. Pathophysiology of ischemia-reperfusion injury. The Journal of Pathology. 2000;**190**:255-266

[91] Bonanno FG. Clinical pathology of the shock syndromes. Journal of Emergencies, Trauma, and Shock. 2011;**4**:233-235

[92] Bonanno FG. Physiopathology of shock. Journal of Emergencies, Trauma, and Shock. 2011;**4**(2):222-232. DOI: 10.4103/0974-2700.82210

[93] Wu MY, Yiang GT, Liao WT, Tsai AP, Cheng YL, Cheng PW, et al. Current

mechanistic concepts in ischemia and reperfusion injury. Cellular Physiology and Biochemistry. 2018;**46**:1650-1667

[94] Douzinas EE, Andrianakis I, Livaditi O, Paneris P, Tasoulis M, Pelekanou A, et al. The level of hypotension during hemorrhagic shock is a major determinant of the post-resuscitation systemic inflammatory response: An experimental study. BMC Physiology. 2008;**8**:15

[95] Santibanez-Gallerani AS, Barber AE, Williams SJ, ZhaoB SY, Shires GT. Improved survival with early fluid resuscitation following hemorrhagic shock. World Journal of Surgery. 2001;**25**(5):592-597. DOI: 10.1007/s002680020115

[96] Lee CC, Chang IJ, Yen ZS, Hsu CY, Chen SY, Su CP, et al. Delayed fluid resuscitation in hemorrhagic shock induces proinflammatory cytokine response. Annals of Emergency Medicine. 2007;**49**(1):37-44. DOI: 10.1016/j.annemergmed.2006.05.031

[97] Malinoski DJ, Slater MS, Mullins RJ. Crush injury and rhabdomyolysis. Critical Care Clinics. 2004;**20**(1):171-192. DOI: 10.1016/s0749-0704(03)00091-5

[98] Bonanno FG. Shock - a reappraisal: The holistic approach. Journal of Emergencies, Trauma, and Shock. 2012;**5**(2):167-177. DOI: 10.4103/0974-2700.96487

[99] Deitch EA. Gut-origin sepsis: Evolution of a concept. The Surgeon. 2012;**10**(6):350-356. DOI: 10.1016/j.surge.2012.03.003. Epub 2012 Apr 23

[100] Assimakopoulos SF, Triantos C, Thomopoulos K, Fligou F, Maroulis I, Marangos M, et al. Gut- origin sepsis in the critically ill patient: Pathophysiology and treatment. Infection. 2018;**46**(6):751-760. DOI: 10.1007/s15010-018-1178-5

[101] Bonanno F. Extending damage control philosophy to not-haemorrhagic situations: Implications for a reclassification of shock states. ANZ Journal of Surgery. 2008;**78**:634-637

[102] Pape HC, Moore EE, McKinley T, Sauaia A. Pathophysiology in patients with polytrauma. Injury. 2022;**53**(7):2400-2412

[103] Callcut RA, Kornblith LZ, Conroy AS, Robles AJ, Meizoso JP, Namias N, et al. The why and how our trauma patients die: A prospective Multicenter Western trauma association study. Journal of Trauma and Acute Care Surgery. 2019;**86**(5):864-870. DOI: 10.1097/TA.0000000000002205

[104] Minei JP, Cuschieri J, Sperry J, Moore EE, West MA, Harbrecht BG, et al. Inflammation and the host response to injury collaborative research program. The changing pattern and implications of multiple organ failure after blunt injury with hemorrhagic shock. Critical Care Medicine. 2012;**40**(4):1129-1135. DOI: 10.1097/CCM.0b013e3182376e9f

[105] Efron P, Brakenridge SC, Mohr AM, Barrios EL, Polcz VE, Anton S, et al. The persistent inflammation, immunosuppression, and catabolism syndrome (PICS) ten years later. Journal of Trauma and Acute Care Surgery. 2023;**95**(5):790-799. DOI: 10.1097/TA.0000000000004087

[106] Douzinas EE. Hemorrhagic shock resuscitation: A critical issue on the development of post- traumatic multiple organ failure. Critical Care Medicine. 2012;**40**:1348-1349

[107] Tachon G, Harrois A, Tanaka S, Kato H, Huet O, Pottecher J. Microcirculatory alterations in traumatic hemorrhagic shock. Critical Care Medicine. 2014;**42**:1433-1441

[108] Ince C. Hemodynamic coherence and rationale for monitoring the microcirculation. Critical Care. 2015;**19**(Suppl. 3):S8

[109] Libert N, Harrois A, Duranteau J. Haemodynamic coherence in haemorrhagic shock. Best Practice & Research. Clinical Anaesthesiology. 2016;**30**:429-435

[110] Bonanno FG. Management of hemorrhagic shock: Physiology approach, timing and strategies. Journal of Clinical Medicine. 2022;**12**:260. DOI: 10.3390/jcm12010260

[111] Bonanno FG. Debunking the lethal triad and delineating damage control surgery. Minerva Surgery. Dec 2023;**78**(6):692-709. DOI: 10.23736/S2724-5691.23.09916-1. Epub 2023 Sep 13

[112] De Backer D, Ospina-Tascon G, Salgado D, Favory R, Creteur J, Vincent J-L. Monitoring the microcirculation in the critically ill patient: Current methods and future approaches. Intensive Care Medicine. 2010;**36**:1813-1825

[113] De Backer D, Donadello K, Sakr Y, Ospina-Tascon G, Salgado D, Colletta S. Microcirculatory alterations in patients with severe sepsis: Impact of time of assessment and relationship with outcome. Critical Care Medicine. 2013;**41**:791-799

[114] Jobsis FF. Noninvasive, infrared monitoring of cerebral and myocardial oxygen sufficiency and circulatory parameters. Science. 1977;**198**(4323):1264-1267

[115] Creteur J, De Backer D, Sakr Y, Koch M. Sublingual capnometry tracks microcirculatory changes in septic patients. Intensive Care Medicine. 2006;**32**:516-523

[116] Heringlake M, Garbers C, Kabler JH, Anderson I, Heinze H, Schon J, et al. Preoperative cerebral oxygen saturation and clinical outcomes in cardiac surgery. Anesthesiology. 2011;**114**(1):58-69

[117] Duret J, Pottecher J, Bouzat P, Brun J, Harrois A, Payen JF, et al. Skeletal muscle oxygenation in severe trauma patients during haemorrhagic shock resuscitation. Critical Care. 2015;**19**:141

[118] Hunt MF, Clark KT, Whitman G, Choi CW, Geocadin RG, Cho SM. The use of cerebral NIRS monitoring to identify acute brain injury in patients with VA-ECMO. Journal of Intensive Care Medicine. 2021;**36**(12):1403-1409

[119] Mayevsky A, Rogatsky GG. Mitochondrial function in vivo evaluated by NADH fluorescence: From animal models to human studies. American Journal of Physiology. Cell Physiology. 2007;**292**(2):C615-C640

[120] Hilty MP, Ince C. Automated quantification of tissue red blood cell perfusion as a new resuscitation target. Current Opinion in Critical Care. 2020;**26**(3):273-280

[121] Hilty MP, Akin S, Boerma C, Donati A, Erdem O, Giaccaglia P, et al. Automated algorithm analysis of sublingual microcirculation in an international multicentral database identifies alterations associated with disease and mechanism of resuscitation. Critical Care Medicine. 2020;**48**:e864-e875

[122] Duranteau J, De Backer D, Donadello K, et al. The future of intensive care: The study of the microcirculation will help to guide our therapies. Critical Care. 2023;**27**:190

[123] Shoemaker WC, Appel PL, Kram HB. Role of oxygen debt in the development of organ failure sepsis, and death in high-risk surgical patients. Chest. 1992;**102**(1):208-215

[124] Fiddian-Green RG, Haglund U, Gutierrez G, Shoemaker WC. Goals for the resuscitation of shock. Critical Care Medicine. 1993;**21**(2 Suppl.):S25-S31

[125] Kipnis E, Vallet B. Early norepinephrine resuscitation of life-threatening hypotensive septic shock: It can do the job, but at what cost? Critical Care. 2010;**14**:450

[126] Cauwels A, Brouckaert P. Nitrite regulation of shock. Cardiovascular Research. 2011;**89**:553-559

[127] Den Uil CA, Caliskan K, Lagrand WK, van der Ent M, Jewbali LS, van Kuijk JP, et al. Dose-dependent benefit of nitroglycerin on microcirculation of patients with severe heart failure. Intensive Care Medicine. 2009;**35**:1893-1899

[128] Tsai AG, Intaglietta M. Exogenous nitric oxide induces protection during hemorrhagic shock. Resuscitation. 2009;**80**:707-712

[129] Cabrales P. Low dose nitrite enhances perfusion after fluid resuscitation from hemorrhagic shock. Resuscitation. 2009;**80**:1431-1436

[130] Nachuraju P, Friedman AJ, Friedman JM, Cabrales P. Exogenous nitric oxide prevents cardiovascular collapse during hemorrhagic shock. Resuscitation. 2011;**82**:607-613

[131] Wang Y, You G, Kan X, Chen G, Zhao L, Zhou H. Nitric oxide inhalation, a proposed strategy for early treatment of hemorrhagic shock. Medical Hypotheses. 2011;**77**:182-184

[132] Samana CM, Diaby M, Fellahi JM, Mdhafar M, Eyraud D, Arock A, et al. Inhibition of platelets aggregation by inhaled nitric oxide in patients with acute respiratory distress syndrome. Anesthesiology. 1995;**83**:56-65

[133] Bloomfield GL, Holloway S, Ridings PC, Fisher BJ, Blocher CR, Sholley M, et al. Pretreatment with inhaled nitric oxide inhibits neutrophil migration and oxidative activity, resulting in attenuated sepsis-induced acute lung injury. Critical Care Medicine. 1997;**25**:584-593

[134] Waisman D, Brod V, Dickstein R, Abramovich A, Rotschild A, Bitterman H. Effects of inhaled nitric oxide on lung injury after intestinal ischemia-reperfusion in rats. Shock. 2005;**23**:150-155

[135] Hines IN, Grisham MB. Divergent roles of superoxide and nitric oxide in liver ischemia and reperfusion injury. Journal of Clinical Biochemistry and Nutrition. 2011;**48**:50-56

[136] Leeper CM, Yazer MH, Cladis FP, Saladino R, Triulzi DJ, Gaines BA. Cold-stored whole blood platelet function is preserved in injured children with hemorrhagic shock. Journal of Trauma and Acute Care Surgery. 2019;**87**(1):49-53

[137] Hazelton JP, Cannon JW, Zatorski C, Roman JS, Moore SA, Young AJ, et al. Cold-stored whole blood: A better method of trauma resuscitation? Journal of Trauma and Acute Care Surgery. 2019;**87**(5):1035-1041

[138] Assen S, Cardenas J, George M, Wang YW, Wade CE, Meyer D, et al. Hemostatic potential of cold-stored non-leukoreduced whole blood over time: An assessment of platelet function and thrombin generation for optimal shelf life. Journal of Trauma and Acute Care Surgery. 2020;**89**:429-434

[139] Clements T, McCoy C, Assen S, Cardenas J, Wade C, Meyer D, et al. The prehospital use of younger age whole blood is associated with an improved

arrival coagulation profile. Journal of Trauma and Acute Care Surgery. 2021;**90**(4):607-614

[140] Fecher A, Stimpson A, Ferrigno L, Pohlman TH. The pathophysiology and management of hemorrhagic shock in the poly-trauma patient. Journal of Clinical Medicine. 2021;**10**:479

[141] Ichikawa J, Kouta M, Oogushi M, Komori M. Effects of room temperature and cold storage on the metabolic and haemostatic properties of whole blood for acute normovolaemic haemodilution. PLoS One. 2022;**17**(5):e0267980

[142] Yanagawa Y, Sakamoto T, Okada Y. Therapeutic hypothermia limited to the resuscitation period does not prolong survival after severe hemorrhagic shock in rats. Resuscitation. 2005;**67**:119-126

[143] Wang P, Cioffi WG, Bland KI, Chaudry IH. Should normothermia be restored and maintained during resuscitation after trauma and hemorrhage? The Journal of Trauma. 2000;**48**:58-65

[144] Takasu A, Norio H, Gotoh Y, Sakamoto T, Okada Y. Effect of induced-hypothermia on short-term survival after volume-controlled hemorrhage in pigs. Resuscitation. 2003;**56**:319-328

[145] Douzinas EE. Progressive hemorrhage: Administer oxygen or early resuscitation? Intensive Care Medicine. 2009;**35**:1664-1666

[146] Murry C, Richard V, Reimer K, Jennings RB. Ischemic preconditioning slows energy metabolism and delays ultrastructural damage during sustained ischemia. Circulation Research. 1990;**66**:913-993

[147] Zhao ZQ, Corvera JS, Halkos ME, Kerendi F, Wang NP, Guyton RA, et al. Inhibition of myocardial injury by ischemic postconditioning during reperfusion: Comparison with ischemic preconditioning. American Journal of Physiology. Heart and Circulatory Physiology. 2003;**285**(2):mH579-88

[148] Crimi G, Pica S, Raineri C, Bramucci E, De Ferrari GM, Klersy C, et al. Remote ischemic post-conditioning of the lower limb during primary percutaneous coronary intervention safely reduces enzymatic infarct size in anterior myocardial infarction: A randomized controlled trial. JACC Cardiovascular Interventions. 2013;**6**(10):1055-1063

[149] Tasoulis MK, Livaditi O, Stamatakos M, Stefanaki C, Paneris P, Prigouris P, et al. High concentrations of reactive oxygen species in the BAL fluid are correlated with lung injury in rabbits after hemorrhagic shock and resuscitation. The Tohoku Journal of Experimental Medicine. 2009;**219**(3):193-1999. DOI: 10.1620/tjem.219.193

[150] Sun HY, Wang NP, Kerendi F, Halkos M, Kin H, Guyton RA, et al. Hypoxic postconditioning reduces cardiomyocyte loss by inhibiting ROS generation and intracellular Ca2+ overload. American Journal of Physiology Heart and Circulatory Physiology. 2005;**288**(4):H1900-H1908

[151] Douzinas EE, Livaditi O, Andrianakis I, Prigouris P, Paneris P, Villiotou V, et al. The effect of hypoxemic resuscitation from hemorrhagic shock on blood pressure restoration and on oxidative and inflammatory responses. Intensive Care Medicine. 2008;**34**:1133-1141

[152] Douzinas EE, Orfanos SE, Livaditi O, Augustatou K, Villiotou V, Kavantzas N, et al. Hypoxemic resuscitation prevents pulmonary

capillary endothelial dysfunction induced by normoxemic resuscitation from hemorrhagic shock. Critical Care Medicine. 2009;**37**:869-875

[153] Younkin DP, Wagerle LC, Chance B, Maria J, Delivoria-Papadopoulos M. 31P-NMR studies of cerebral metabolic changes during graded hypoxia in newborn lambs. Journal of Applied Physiology. 1987;**62**(4):1569-1574

[154] Tasoulis MK, Douzinas EE. Hypoxemic reperfusion of ischemic states: An alternative approach for the attenuation of oxidative stress mediated reperfusion injury. Journal of Biomedical Science. 2016;**23**:7. DOI: 10.1186/s12929-016-0220-0

[155] Dyson A, Stidwill R, Taylor V, Singer M. The impact of inspired oxygen concentration on tissue oxygenation during progressive haemorrhage. Intensive Care Medicine. 2009;**35**:1783-1791

[156] Hafner C, Wu J, Tiboldi A, Hess M, Mitulovic G, Kaun C, et al. Hyperoxia induces inflammation and cytotoxicity in human adult cardiac myocytes. Shock. 2017;**47**:436-444

[157] Muller CR, Courelli V, Govender K, Omert L, Yoshida T, Cabrales P. Hypoxically stored RBC resuscitation in a rat model of traumatic brain injury and severe hemorrhagic shock. Life Sciences. 2024;**340**:122423. DOI: 10.1016/j.lfs.2024.122423

[158] Naumann DN, Hazeldine J, Midwinter MJ, Hutchings SD, Harrison P. Poor microcirculatory flow dynamics are associated with endothelial cell damage and glycocalyx shedding after traumatic hemorrhagic shock. Journal of Trauma and Acute Care Surgery. 2018;**84**:81-88

[159] Cardenas J, Dong JF, Kozar RA. Injury-induced endotheliopathy: What you need to know. Journal of Trauma and Acute Care Surgery. 2023;**95**(4):454-463

[160] Milford EM, Reade MC. Resuscitation fluid choices to preserve the endothelial Glycocalyx. Critical Care. 2019;**23**:77

[161] Reitz KM, Moore HB, Guyette FX, Sauaia A, Pusateri AE, Moore EE, et al. Prehospital plasma in injured patients is associated with survival principally in blunt injury: Results from two randomized prehospital plasma trials. Journal of Trauma and Acute Care Surgery. 2020;**88**(1):33-41. DOI: 10.1097/TA.0000000000002485

[162] Diebel LN, Liberati DM. Effect of tranexamic acid on endothelial von Willebrand factor/ADAMTS-13 response to in vitro shock conditions. Journal of Trauma and Acute Care Surgery. 2023;**94**(2):273-280

[163] Bitterman H. Bench-to-bedside review: Oxygen as a drug. Critical Care. 2009;**13**(1):205

[164] Weenink RP, de Jonge SW, van Hulst RA, Wingelaar TT, van Ooij PAM, Immink RV, et al. Perioperative hyperoxyphobia: Justified or not? Benefits and harms of hyperoxia during surgery. Journal of Clinical Medicine. 2020;**9**:642

[165] Hunt TK. Normal repair. In: Hunt TK, Dunphy JE, editors. Fundamentals of Wound Management. New York: Appleton Century Crofts; 1979. pp. 53-63

[166] Hunt TK. Disorders of repair and their management. In: Hunt TK, Dunphy JE, editors. Fundamentals of Wound Management. New York: Appleton Century Crofts; 1979. pp. 96-103

[167] Gutierrez G, Marini C, Acero AL, Lund N. Skeletal muscle PO2 during

hypoxemia and isovolemic anemia. Journal of Applied Physiology (1985). 1990;**68**(5):2047-2053. DOI: 10.1152/jappl.1990.68.5.2047

[168] Aggarwal NR, Brower RG, Hager DN, Thompson BT, Netzer G, Shanholtz C, et al. Oxygen exposure resulting in arterial oxygen tensions above the protocol goal was associated with worse clinical outcomes in acute respiratory distress syndrome. Critical Care Medicine. 2018;**46**(4):517-524

[169] Convertino VA, Lye KR, Koons NJ, Joyner MJ. Physiological comparison of hemorrhagic shock and VO_2max: A conceptual framework for defining the limitation of oxygen delivery. Experimental Biology and Medicine (Maywood, N.J.). 2019;**244**(8):690-701

Chapter 6

Enhanced Recovery after Surgery (ERAS) in Emergency and Trauma Surgery

Ruggero Bollino, Helen Yu, Davide Luppi and Maurizio Zizzo

Abstract

Enhanced Recovery After Surgery (ERAS) protocols reduce the length of hospital stay (LHS), complications, and costs for many elective surgical procedures. The ERAS protocol concerns a multimodal, multidisciplinary, standardized, evidence-based approach to minimize stress for patients undergoing surgery. A similar, structured approach appears to improve outcomes, including mortality, for patients undergoing high-risk emergency general surgery, and emergency laparotomy, in particular. Recently, several studies have been published, including new guidelines, analyzing the benefits of ERAS protocols in emergency surgery and trauma patients. The aim of this chapter is to analyze the available data and the benefits of using ERAS protocols in patients undergoing emergency and trauma surgery.

Keywords: enhanced recovery after surgery, emergency, trauma, surgery, protocol

1. Introduction

Originating from the pioneering work of Professor Henrik Kehlet in the 1990s at the University of Copenhagen, Denmark, the Enhanced Recovery After Surgery (ERAS) protocol concerns a multimodal, multidisciplinary, standardized, evidence-based approach to minimize stress for patients undergoing surgery, promoting healthy organ function, and ultimately improving outcomes [1]. The first guidelines, developed by the ERAS Study Group, founded in 2001 by Professor Ken Fearon of the University of Edinburgh, UK, and Professor Olle Ljungqvist of the Karolinska Institutet, Sweden, focused on patients undergoing colorectal surgery [2]. Subsequently, in 2009, guidelines for implementation of enhanced recovery protocols (ERPs) were published by the Association of Surgeons of Great Britain and Ireland (ASGBI) [3]. These guidelines, which involve surgeons, anesthetists, nurses, and allied health professionals, address pre-admission, pre-operative, intra-operative, and post-operative items. It was demonstrated that adherence to each component of the ERAS protocol can significantly reduce length of hospital stay (LHS), infection risks, complications such as anastomotic leak, and overall morbidity and mortality rates [4–6].

 IntechOpen

2. Principles of ERAS protocol

Pre-operative optimization for elective surgery requires treating modifiable medical conditions like diabetes, hypertension, renal disease, atrial fibrillation, chronic obstructive pulmonary disease (COPD), and asthma to achieve optimal patient performance status and minimize related complications. Also, as pre-operative anemia is linked to in-hospital mortality, 30-day mortality, stroke, acute kidney injury, and sepsis [7], oral or intravenous iron therapy or erythropoietin therapy should be assessed to reach a target of hemoglobin (Hb) >12–13 g/dL.

Nutritional assessments are crucial for identifying malnutrition, hyponutrition, and sarcopenia, given their predictive value for mortality, LHS, infections, and anastomotic leaks [8–10]. Appropriate interventions, including oral diets, weight loss, or nutritional support, can reduce complications by approximately 25% [11]. Prehabilitation along with smoking and alcohol cessation was proven to significantly improve patient outcomes [12–15].

Many ERAS items have challenged traditional surgical dogma through an in-depth understanding of the pathophysiological response to surgical stress. For instance, the practice of pre-operative fasting was reevaluated following observations of worsened outcomes in animal models and evidence supporting rapid gastric emptying after fluid intake [16].

Studies comparing patients undergoing intravenous glucose infusion with or without insulin treatment to fasted patients demonstrated improved insulin sensitivity, reduced post-operative protein loss, and lower cortisol level increases after surgery [17, 18]. Following these findings, the ERAS group developed a low-osmolarity carbohydrate-rich drink (maltodextrin) to improve gastric emptying and stimulate the insulin response [19].

Pre-operative bowel preparation before colorectal surgery was questioned due to the potential risks of hypovolemia and electrolyte imbalance, which can worsen cardiac or renal comorbidities. Studies indicated that bowel preparation may exacerbate post-operative ileus and affect anastomotic healing. As a result, bowel preparation was discouraged and rectal enemas are suggested as the preferred approach for left colon and rectal surgery [20].

Careful attention by the anesthesiologist is required during intra-operative management, particularly with regard to antimicrobial prophylaxis, prevention of hypothermia, monitoring of the depth of anesthesia and neuromuscular blockade, intravenous fluid management, and analgesia.

Hypothermia was proven to increase blood loss (16%) requiring blood transfusion (22%), increased stress response with excessive catecholamine release causing vasoconstriction, increased afterload, myocardial ischemia, cardiac arrhythmias, surgical site infection, and coagulopathy [21].

Intra-operative fluid management should aim to optimize cardiac function, intravascular volume, and tissue perfusion with an appropriate near-zero balance line [22]. Excessive fluid administration may result in pulmonary and anastomotic edema. Conversely, inadequate fluid intake can reduce cardiac output. Poor fluid management is also associated with increased inflammatory and metabolic markers such as interleukin 6 (IL-6) and reactive oxygen species (ROS) during a major surgery [23]. Goal-directed fluid therapy is recommended by ERAS guidelines.

Monitoring the depth of anesthesia and maintaining neuromuscular blockade enable the effective management of general anesthetic drugs and the prevention of cognitive dysfunction and post-operative delirium [24].

Multimodal analgesia, tailored to the surgical approach, is essential. Whenever possible, offering minimally invasive surgery (MIS) along with multimodal analgesia is recommended. Inadequate analgesic programs can exacerbate surgical stress, leading to poor mobilization, prolonged bed rest, respiratory issues, and delayed gastrointestinal function return, thereby prolonging hospital stay [21]. A balance of good anesthesia, stress response modification, and satisfactory side effect profile should be achieved [21].

Epidural anesthesia should be avoided due to their potential to alter endocrine and metabolic responses to surgical stress. Patient-controlled analgesia (PCA) has been associated with high pain scores in the early post-operative period, indicating inadequate pain control. Opioid-sparing analgesia should be assessed to avoid post-operative nausea and vomiting and delayed gastrointestinal function return. Minimal opioid use in the shortest period, combined with anti-inflammatory steroidal and non-steroidal drugs, plays a key role in managing surgical stress and inflammation. Initially, spinal analgesia was considered preferable to epidurals and PCA because it allowed for opioid-sparing therapies. However, the introduction of abdominal wall blocks demonstrated similar outcomes in MIS while avoiding the side effect of hypotension and offering the added benefits of rapid awakening and early mobilization [25].

The ERAS program does not promote a particular minimally invasive technique, but instead advocates for avoiding open surgery as it has been shown to be an independent factor in improving outcomes, reducing LHS, avoiding wound complications such as surgical site infections and incisional hernias, and minimizing stress responses [4, 26]. **Table 1** illustrates the impact of fast-track care versus standard care on the length of hospital stay in colonic surgery [27]:

Two other frequently debated items concern the use of drains and the nasogastric tube. In ERAS, the routine use of drainage should be avoided as they can act as a foreign body, potentially providing a pathway for contamination, and are often rapidly obstructed and therefore ineffective. Drains should be reserved for selected high-risk patients and removed early [28].

The use of nasogastric tube has been challenged as well, as it is ineffective for its purpose of decreasing gastric distension after surgery and avoiding respiratory complications such as pneumonia and pulmonary aspiration. Multiple systematic reviews of randomized trials have shown that patients who do not undergo routine nasogastric tube decompression or receive "early tube removal" experience a faster return of bowel function and reduced pulmonary complications compared to those who kept it in place until intestinal function had returned. Furthermore, some studies demonstrated an opposite effect on intestinal function return of gastric tube and pharyngeal and respiratory adverse events [29]. In upper gastrointestinal surgery, no difference in anastomotic leakage and mortality has been demonstrated in routine nasogastric decompression versus early removal, or in nasogastric tube reinsertion [30, 31].

The most innovative features of the ERAS protocol can be found in the post-operative management.

LHS in colonic surgery	Fast-track care	Standard of care
Laparoscopic surgery	5 (4–7) days	6 (4–8.5) days
Open surgery	6 (4.5–10) days	7 (6–10.5) days

Table 1.
Results from Enroll (enhanced recovery open versus laparoscopic): A multicenter randomized trial of conventional versus laparoscopic surgery for colorectal cancer within an enhanced recovery program [27].

Early oral feeding has been shown to be safe: no increase in relevant complications was observed, and yet a decrease in mortality was observed when started within 24 h of surgery [32]. Functional recovery, major complications, and LHS were reduced in patients who were able to tolerate normal food from the first day even after gastrointestinal surgery [33]. Enteral nutrition supplementation in selected cases is necessary. Controversial results have been seen with immunonutrition: some trials showed a significant reduction in infectious complications [34, 35]. As oral intake starts quickly, intravenous fluid therapies should be taken into account only as supplement when oral intake is not sufficient, in order to avoid edema [33].

Early removal of the urinary catheter is another important challenge of the ERAS protocol, which promotes early mobilization and contributes to the prevention of post-operative ileus, which is another important goal [5].

Post-operative ileus is the consequence of a disturbance of neuronal and hormonal balance which creates a disorganized electrical activity and paralysis of the bowel [36].

Enhanced Recovery After Surgery (ERAS) items in colorectal surgery (2018)
1. Pre-admission information, education, counseling
2. Pre-operative optimization
3. Prehabilitation
4. Pre-operative nutritional care
5. Management of anemia
6. Prevention of nausea and vomiting (PONV)
7. Pre-anesthetic medication
8. Antimicrobial prophylaxis and skin preparation
9. Bowel preparation
10. Pre-operative fluid and electrolyte therapy
11. Pre-operative fasting and carbohydrate loading
12. Standard anesthetic protocol
13. Intra-operative fluid and electrolyte therapy
14. Preventing intra-operative hypothermia
15. Surgical access (open vs. minimal invasive surgery)
16. Drainage of peritoneal cavity and pelvis
17. Nasogastric intubation
18. Multimodal post-operative analgesia
19. Thromboprophylaxis
20. Post-operative fluid and electrolyte therapy
21. Urinary catheter
22. Prevention of post-operative ileus
23. Post-operative glycemic control
24. Post-operative nutritional care
25. Early mobilization

Table 2.
Guidelines for perioperative Care in Elective Colorectal Surgery: Enhanced recovery after surgery (ERAS) society recommendations [5].

Reducing edema, controlling electrolytes and the inflammatory response, sparing opioids, using minimally invasive surgery (MIS), avoiding the nasogastric tube, and implementing early feeding and mobilization can prevent post-operative ileus [37]. Prokinetics and laxatives can be used to treat it.

Antimicrobial prophylaxis should be given once before surgery. If contamination happens during surgery, it may be necessary to extend prophylaxis up to 24 h. Empirical treatment should be considered if the surgical site is contaminated and administered for a maximum of 3–5 days or as per the specific case. Long-term use of antibiotics is related to severe infections caused by antibiotic-resistant bacteria, which can lead to a higher mortality rate [38].

Prophylaxis for thromboembolism should be assessed based on risk factors and should be balanced against risk of bleeding. Pharmacological and non-pharmacological treatments should be used based on the risk assessment and for no longer than 14 days in ERAS protocol. Oral anticoagulant should be reintroduced as soon as the risk of bleeding is negligible (**Table 2**) [5].

Based on this evidence, many studies conducted worldwide demonstrated the feasibility of ERAS protocols and significant reduction in complications and post-operative mortality in these patients [39–41].

The ERAS protocol has faced criticism regarding readmission issues due to early discharge. However, the ERAS pathway does not compromise the standard of care's fundamental principle of "safety first" but rather adds an efficiency perspective, challenging dogmatic questions and focusing on prehabilitation. Data have shown a decreased LHS without impact on readmission and emergency room utilization [42].

As the results became clearer, each side of surgery started to tailor its own protocol, adapting items for each situation. There are very few studies on trauma because of the disruptive nature of the emergency environment.

3. Enhanced recovery protocols in emergency surgery

The convincing results obtained in colorectal surgery led to investigating this kind of protocol in emergency surgery as well.

Among the earliest studies, convincing evidence of the effectiveness of ERPs in emergency surgery was provided by three landmark studies.

Møller et al.'s study evaluated the effect of a multimodal, multidisciplinary perioperative care program on mortality in patients with perforated peptic ulcers across seven Danish hospitals. The implementation of this program resulted in a remarkable reduction of 37% in the 30-day mortality rate compared to historical and concurrent national controls. This translates to saving one life for every 10 patients treated [43].

In the NELA (National Emergency Laparotomy Audit) study, the introduction of an emergency laparotomy pathway quality improvement care (ELPQuIC) bundle across four UK hospitals significantly reduced the risk of death following emergency laparotomy [44]. The ELPQuIC bundle encompassed a comprehensive set of evidence-based interventions, including early warning scores, early antibiotics, prompt surgery, goal-directed hemodynamic therapy, and post-operative intensive care. Because of implementation of this care bundle, the number of lives saved per 100 patients treated increased from 6.47 to 12.44. Remarkably, this improvement in mortality was observed without any significant difference in patient severity as assessed by the Portsmouth-Physiological and Operative Severity Score for the Enumeration of Mortality and Morbidity (P-POSSUM).

A subsequent study further examined the economic implications of implementing the ELPQuIC bundle, considering both hospital and societal perspectives. The analysis, conducted in accordance with the Consolidated Health Economic Evaluation Reporting Standards (CHEERS) guidelines, revealed that while in-hospital costs were slightly higher, societal costs were reduced overall. This highlights the potential for cost savings to healthcare systems through the adoption of this care bundle [45].

The first evaluation of the ERAS pathway in emergency surgery focused on obstructive colorectal cancer treated in an emergency setting [46]. Lohsiriwat et al. published in 2014 the first retrospective comparison between standard of care and ERAS pathway for these patients, demonstrating its safety and beneficial effects. There were no differences in mortality or readmission between the groups, but the ERAS group started oral nutrition earlier, with an earlier return of bowel function and a shorter LHS, which meant an earlier start to adjuvant chemotherapy.

The first randomized study on applying ERAS program components after emergency surgery was published in 2014 by Gonenc et al. from Turkey for peptic ulcer perforation [47]. This landmark study demonstrated the feasibility and safety of implementing ERAS principles in the emergency setting. The study compared the outcomes of patients undergoing emergency laparotomy for peptic ulcer perforation who received either a standard care protocol or an ERAS-modified protocol and found that patients who received the ERAS-modified protocol had significantly shorter LHS, quicker return to oral intake, and lower rates of post-operative complications compared to those who received standard care. These findings highlighted the potential of ERAS to improve patient outcomes even in the context of emergency surgery.

Quiney et al. in 2016 identified key areas for improvement in the ERAS pathway for emergency settings [48]. They observed that delays in diagnosis could lead to delays and inadequate resuscitation, sepsis assessment, and post-operative care when intensive care unit (ICU) stay is needed. To address these issues, they proposed a stepwise approach that focuses on accelerating diagnosis in cases of ambiguous symptoms, early administration of broad-spectrum antibiotics after sepsis assessment, and predicting ICU stay.

Wisely et al. highlighted a changing mindset in their Australian group in the post-ERAS era (2016) [49]. They observed how ERAS principles had influenced their management in emergency surgery as a natural evolution of their pre-ERAS conventional care. For example, intravenous fluid infusion decreased sensitively after ERAS guidelines' publication for elective surgery ($p < 0.001$), urinary catheter was considered unnecessary for more than 2 days and removed earlier in post-ERAS ($p < 0.001$), earlier removal of PCA has been seen ($p = 0.001$) and reduced drain placement ($p = 0.001$). No differences were seen between the two periods for anastomosis or stoma, oral intake, nasogastric tube use or earlier removal. Less major complications were observed in the post-ERAS group ($p = 0.002$) and when present they were related, on a multivariate analysis, to an important ERAS statement, which is an unfulfilled fluid balance within the first 48 h. At the end of their description, the group was enthusiastic about promoting other challenging principles of the ERAS protocols in emergency surgery.

Randomized trial with the aim of applying more ERAS items on emergency surgery was published with convincing results [50]. As experiences grew, other pathologies than intestinal obstruction and peptic ulcer perforation were treated with ERAS program highlighting the differences with elective surgery and the limited compliance, for example, in case of intra-abdominal infections [51].

The Spanish study by Viñas et al. showed the safety and benefit of ERAS-adapted program in left colectomy after colonic perforation. The new management showed significantly lower morbidity rates, with no additional mortality or readmissions. The ERAS group also showed a significantly shorter LHS. Their conclusion was that the ERAS guidelines should implement the emergency setting [52].

The key difference between emergency and elective surgery patients is that the former presents in a compromised state, often in high-risk patients with systemic inflammatory response syndrome (SIRS), sepsis or shock. The outcomes in emergency surgery are poor, with higher risk of death up to one-tenth at 30 days after surgery, one-fourth for patient over the age of 80 years, and higher risk of complications [53].

The above fact has been underlined by the encouraging results of several recent narrative reviews, systematic reviews, and meta-analyses on this topic [54–60].

4. ERAS principles in emergency surgery

Enhanced Recovery After Surgery (ERAS) Society finally published its own guidelines for perioperative care for emergency laparotomy in 2021 and 2023, including all the abdominal non-elective procedures, potentially life-threatening, excluding trauma laparotomies, vascular procedures, appendectomy, and cholecystectomy [61].

Pre-operative management is very different from elective surgery, and the main aim is to promptly correct any alteration in the patient's homeostasis during investigations and diagnosis. Resuscitation and Early Warning Score (EWS) should guide a stepwise system of care: circulatory and respiratory stabilization, early goal-directed fluid therapy, and minimization of surgical delay have been shown by many studies to reduce mortality and LHS after surgery in this setting [62–64].

The pathophysiological derangement, such as SIRS or sepsis, gut dysfunction, insulin resistance, fluid shifts, and many others, depending on patient's comorbidities and performance status, may last longer than its presentation. This may be considered for the treatment and the goal result [61]. Risk assessment using validated scores should guide pathways of care, whether non-operative management or operative one [65, 66].

Patient with multiple-organ failure (MOF) presentation, requiring damage-control surgery with open abdomen or ICU post-operative stay longer than 72 h, should not be candidate to ERAS protocol [61].

In these cases, the speed and efficiency of the process should be increased: in the first hour, blood cultures should be obtained, antibiotics should be promptly assessed, resuscitation with crystalloid should be evaluated and monitored by blood lactate, and potential vasopressors started [67].

Rapid diagnosis and treatment planning should be made: every delay is a cost to the patient survival, complications, and prolonged LHS. Computed tomography (CT) scan with intravenous contrast medium is the gold standard for abdominal diagnosis and should be acquired and discussed between surgeon and radiologist as soon as possible, whenever the patient is stable. In case of sepsis, the source control should be achieved surgically or through interventional radiology within 3 h from admission if shock is present, 6 h if not [61]. A Danish study proved that delayed emergency surgery in perforated peptic ulcer leads to reduced survival for every hour of delay from hospital admission [68], while a British study based on National Emergency Laparotomy Audit (NELA) data showed an increased mortality for delay beyond 72 h [69].

Pre-operative multidisciplinary counseling to the patient and the patient's family with detailed information about the procedure, potential complication with stepwise strategies and post-operative pathway should be assessed, and most importantly, shared decision-making plays a crucial role in an emergency setting for a potentially fatal event [70].

The evaluation of frailty and cognitive assessment must be undertaken in elderly patients to optimize post-operative care, avoiding perioperative neurocognitive disorders and delirium triggered by medications [61]. The use of benzodiazepines should be avoided in elderly patients for the potential trigger to delirium and opioids should be minimized to avoid oversedation and hypoventilation [71].

In a patient who takes antithrombotic medications, reversal agents can be used prior emergency surgery to reduce the risk of hemorrhage. Vitamin K, fresh frozen plasma, prothrombin complex concentrate (PCC), recombinant coagulation factor, and monoclonal antibodies (idarucizumab) should be used if any major surgery is to be performed. Consider platelet transfusion in patients on antiplatelet therapy, after evaluation by a cardiologist, if there's is a history of a recent coronary stent or procedure [72].

Fluid management should be goal directed, avoiding patient overload even in case of severe hypotension where inotropes can help to sustain circulation [61]. Electrolyte disorders (hypokalemia, hypomagnesemia, and hypophosphatemia) are frequent, potentially a trigger for atrial fibrillation, and should be corrected before or during surgery.

Hyperglycemia is also very common for the high levels of cortisol release, particularly in diabetic patients, but it leads to an overproduction of inflammatory mediators, ROS and free fatty acids (FFAs), which are potentially harmful to the endothelial vascular compartment and the immune system and can cause cellular damage [73].

There is no need to prepare the patient with carbohydrate load as in elective surgery, instead correction with insulin or glucose to reach levels of 144–180 mg/dL can reduce complications and mortality.

The use of nasogastric tubes in an emergency setting has a different rationale than elective surgery and has a different risk-benefit ratio. Aspiration of gastric distention for high gastric fluids may be beneficial. Post-operative management may be different than elective setting as well [61].

From an anesthesiologist's point of view, emergency surgery patient is more demanding, frequently needs rapid sequence induction and intubation [74] for the higher risk of airway contamination, using fast curare and eventually cricoid compression, monitoring the depth of anesthesia with particular attention to the use of propofol in emergencies due to its hypotensive effects associated with increased use of vasopressors [75]. Ventilation as well should be carefully supervised because of the association between high peak pressure and development of post-operative pulmonary complication [76]. ERAS guidelines on emergency surgery suggest to start with a tidal volume of 6–8 ml/kg and a positive end expiratory pressure (PEEP) of 5 cmH_2O and thereafter to tailor it to patient needs [77].

Indication for neuromuscular block monitoring, PONV reduction, and temperature maintenance are similar to elective ERAS principles.

Multimodal opioid-sparing analgesia may be different and limited in an emergency setting: epidural catheter placement may not be safe in the presence of sepsis and coagulopathic modification, non-steroidal anti-inflammatory drugs (NSAIDs) should be cautiously used because of the high risk of acute kidney injury (AKI) in multiple-organ failure (MOF) patients, paracetamol as well in case of liver failure. Neuraxial blocks should be avoided in hemodynamically unstable patients to avoid sympathetic blockade, vasodilatation, and hypotension [75]. The use of local anesthetics on surgical wound, transversus abdominis plane (TAP) blockade, and intraperitoneal infiltration with local anesthetic could be effective in reducing post-operative pain within the first 6 h and opioid use in the first 24 h [78–81].

Intra-operative choices should be based on the risk/benefit assessment considering not only patient's conditions and pathology but also surgeon's preference, skill, and experience.

Initial diagnostic laparoscopy is recommended because of the benefits already outlined, with an eventual conversion to open laparotomy [75]. If a gastrointestinal or colorectal anastomosis is required, the risk of leakage must be assessed [82, 83]. Even if the emergency setting represents a major risk it should not be considered as a contraindication*per se*, as in many cases a primary anastomosis can be performed safely and should be carefully considered alongside any other alternative strategy [75]. Resection and stoma creation should be assessed in a shocked patient requiring vasopressor support.

In a critically ill patient, damage control for hemorrhage or source of infection control achieved as soon as possible delaying definitive anastomosis and abdominal wall closure for a planned re-laparotomy [84] was challenged in ERAS protocol. Whenever possible, definitive primary anastomosis and abdominal wall closure were demonstrated to lead to fewer overall operations, shorter ICU stay, and total hospital stay [85]. The use of negative pressure wound therapy (NPWT) for abdominal wall closure may be used for intra-abdominal sepsis, to reduce complications, reinterventions, and infections. Deferred wall closure may benefit from dynamic mesh traction on fascia besides vacuum-assisted closure therapy (VAC therapy) [86].

Traditionally, emergency laparotomy claimed routinary drainage, but many studies demonstrated no benefit over such routinary drainage. The World Society of Emergency Surgery (WSES) discouraged the use of drain in perforated appendicitis with or without abscess or peritonitis because there were no benefits about intra-abdominal abscess formation or surgical site infections [87]. Drain-related morbidities were described after perforated peptic ulcer as well (fever, peritoneal fluid collection, surgical site infection, and wound dehiscence) [88].

Antibiotic prophylaxis with a broad-spectrum agent should be administered and continued according to diagnosis, intra-operative findings, and field contamination [89]. Skin antisepsis is recommended. Use of a wound protector, new instruments, and glove change for closure was shown to bring about effective reduction of superficial and deep surgical site of infection [90].

At the end of an emergency procedure, the impact of surgery on metabolic and hemodynamic stability for extubation may be considered. Because of the high risk of re-intubation related to an ASA III patient (i.e., a patient with severe systemic disease as per the American Society of Anethesiologists' (ASA) Physical Status Classification System) and abdominal surgery, frequently occurring in an emergency setting, extubation may not be indicated [91, 92]. A careful assessment of the patient's condition should be scored in order to decide whether to extubate or transfer with intubated patient to the ICU, and patient post-operative destination [75].

In order to prevent post-operative pulmonary complication and facilitate extubation, non-invasive positive-pressure ventilation and continuous positive airway pressure should be used only when the patient presents acute respiratory failure [93]. High flow nasal cannula oxygen is an interesting alternative with lower gastric air aspiration, increasingly used after COVID-19 pandemic era, but not yet investigated after emergency surgery [94].

Post-operative management should be adapted to a patient's condition. Cognitive impairment can be a consequence of MOF, benzodiazepines and anticholinergics should be avoided after delirium and neurocognitive assessment [95]. Mouth care, regular communication to the patient, and sleep hygiene care were demonstrated to reduce delirium [96, 97].

Post-operative thromboprophylaxis with low-molecular-weight heparins should be extended after discharge based on risk assessment, considering emergency surgery as a major risk and including the burden of surgery, malignancy, inflammatory bowel disease, and travel after surgery [98, 99].

In contrast to the ERAS indication in elective surgery, early removal of the urinary catheter cannot be safely achieved in this setting due to the need to monitor fluid balance in the first post-operative days in a life-threatening patient condition [100]. It may also be difficult following pelvic surgery and the resulting immobility, so the possibility of catheter removal should be evaluated daily after the critical period has passed for these patients [101].

With regard to early removal of the nasogastric tube, since the first application of the ERAS program in emergency surgery, its feasibility was demonstrated alongside the benefits of early oral nutrition [47]. In these cases, the nasogastric tube should only be used for therapeutic purposes, such as post-operative ileus or bowel edema at the end of surgery [29].

Early oral feeding was shown to be safe, even after emergency surgery [102, 103], although it is sometimes associated with episodes of mild vomiting and is also a measure to avoid post-operative ileus, in addition to mini-invasive surgery, opioid-sparing analgesia and, most importantly, optimized fluid management.

Enteral nutrition, or even mixed enteral and parenteral nutrition, is a valid alternative if the patient cannot be started on oral nutrition (e.g., if the patient is intubated) and the caloric requirements are not met [104].

Parenteral nutrition should only be started in the event of obstruction, sepsis, intestinal ischemia, high output fistula, or gastrointestinal bleeding. Adequate caloric intake should be achieved in the less invasive way possible.

In summary, rehabilitation is a crucial point to address in the emergency population, as prolonged bed rest, catabolic status worsening potential, pre-existing sarcopenia [105] and insulin resistance are common and associated with poor outcome and higher mortality. Early mobilization is strongly recommended [75].

In the emergency setting, optimization of perioperative care is even more important and, following the publication of the ERAS guidelines for emergency surgery, adherence to the ERAS pathway is even more widely recommended to improve patient outcomes.

The WSES also provided its own indication for the implementation of the ERAS protocol in a recently published position paper [106]. From their perspective, the adherence to enhanced recovery program may improve patient compliance as a chained process, which can result in reduced LHS with no increasing complication and readmission. WSES reinforced ERAS principles, adding their position about antibiotics, which should be continued after surgery for a short course only in case of complicated infections.

Pre-operative optimization is necessary, but the timing of surgery may dictate the speed of re-equilibration: WSES identified the need for a balance between immediate surgery for early resolution of acute illness and delayed surgery for improvement of the patient's condition. The WSES paper highlights another critical issue that relates to the wide heterogeneity of protocols reported in published studies on this topic and the consequent lack of good quality evidence.

Ceresoli et al. first published their experience with a larger population after the ERAS guidelines were published [107]. Their results showed that implementation of the early recovery protocol was feasible and effective, with adherence to the items leading to a shorter LHS and fewer complications, while non-adherence was associated with delayed recovery. On regression analysis, use of laparoscopy was associated with increasing adherence to ERAS principles, whereas a negative effect was seen for the presence of hyperglycemia, fluid overload, drain placement, duration of surgery, and major complication. This study emphasized that the elements of ERAS are interconnected and the lack of one of them can reduce the effectiveness of the whole process. To implement ERAS, the Italian group suggested operative hemodynamic monitoring to reduce fluid infusion and encourage the use of inotropes to maintain the circulatory compartment, discouraged the use of drains in the absence of contamination, and emphasized the importance of pre-operative correction of hyperglycemia and the increasing use of minimally invasive approaches.

5. Enhanced recovery protocols in trauma surgery

As in the emergency setting, applying pre-operative and intra-operative ERAS considerations in trauma surgery presents challenges and limitations. These are due to factors including features' presentation, the need for rapid intervention, surgical risk, and patient pre-existing conditions. However, some of the ERAS principles can potentially improve the outcomes, even in a trauma setting.

There is sparse literature on the implementation of an enhanced recovery program following trauma surgery. ERAS guidelines omit this scenario due to insufficient research and inadequate understanding of improvement areas.

In 2016, Moydien et al. published an analysis of the impact of their study on enhanced recovery after emergency laparotomy for penetrating abdominal trauma. Their protocol included post-operative elements, such as early removal of urinary catheters, nasogastric tubes, and intravenous lines, early oral feeding, analgesia, and early mobilization. The group of patients who received treatment following this protocol was compared to a similar group with comparable injuries who underwent treatment prior to the implementation of the new intervention. The results showed that there was good adherence to the protocol with no significant differences in complications, but patients who underwent ERP had significantly shorter LHS (5.5 ± 1.8 days vs. 8.4 ± 4.2 days, $p < 0.0002$). Although it was a pilot study with small sample, it demonstrated that ERAS principles could be applied effectively and safely in cases of penetrating abdominal trauma [108].

The first randomized controlled trial of ERAS application after trauma surgery was published in 2021 by Purushothaman et al. Multiple items were tested in the ERAS patient group, resulting in a reduction of 1.7 days in LHS (3.3 ± 1.3 days vs. 5 ± 1.7 days, $p < 0.01$) without any differences in complication or readmission. Nonetheless, this study has several limitations. First, the population selection was not comparable to the typical scenario due to the exclusion of ASA III–IV patients. Second, the ERAS milestone indication for goal-directed fluid management was not achieved and excessive amounts of colloids were given, probably resulting in four cases of ERAS failure due to paralytic ileus and vomiting after consuming solid food. On the other hand, the explanation of the trauma dynamics and their correlation with other trauma scenarios, including orthopedic, thoracic, and pelvic injuries, is very interesting in terms of its implications for pre- and post-operative management and the implementation of the ERAS pathway for these patients [109].

Uchino et al. published a scoping review on emergency abdominal surgery and trauma in 2023. They found only four studies on ERP application in the context of trauma, with only two specifically focused on trauma. All four studies aimed to evaluate the efficacy of the enhanced recovery protocol and only one trial looked exclusively at post-operative principles. The analyzed ERP items comprised:

- Pre-operative items: arterial/central line insertion, early prophylactic antibiotics, pre-anesthetic medication, nasogastric intubation, and urinary catheter insertion.

- Intra-operative items: standard anesthetic protocol, goal-directed fluid therapy, multimodal analgesia, prevention of hypothermia, and avoidance of routinary drain placement.

- Post-operative items: post-operative nutritional care, early removal of nasogastric tube, urinary catheter and drain, early mobilization and physiotherapeutic intervention, use of antibiotic, thromboembolism prophylaxis, and prevention of peptic ulcer.

The primary results of the study show a reduction in LHS, early return of bowel function, and early functional recovery using the ERAS principles. Importantly, there were no significant differences in complication rates.

Nevertheless, the authors outlined a number of issues that need to be considered in the implementation of ERAS protocols in these patients, including: necessity to manage trauma in a high-volume center with a dedicated trauma system and multidisciplinary team, high heterogeneity of the patient population and of baseline comorbidities (trauma patients vary greatly in the severity of their injuries) ranging from minor to severe trauma, a wide range of procedure complexities (trauma laparotomies cover a range of procedures from simple bowel resections to more demanding damage-control procedures) [58].

6. Conclusions

Current literature has shown that following ERAS guidelines leads to excellent outcomes in reducing post-operative complications and mortality in a wide range of elective general surgical scenarios.

Although recent studies provided good results about the possibility of reducing post-operative non-surgical and surgical complications and LHS through the application of ERAS protocols, their implementation in the context of emergency surgery may face different challenges. In particular, some aforementioned challenges are urgency/emergency of care, severity of the primary pathology requiring emergency treatment, heterogeneity of patient populations (e.g., comorbidities) and procedures, availability of resources, and the need for dedicated and highly specialized professionals (e.g., surgeons, anesthetists, ICU physicians, and nurses).

To date, the real evidence about the benefits of applying ERAS principles in emergency and trauma surgery is poor. Therefore, it appears necessary to conduct further well-designed randomized controlled trials, possibly multicenter ones, in order to confirm or not the positive results coming from the few existing studies, mainly observational ones. However, the feasibility of studies with designs having greater statistical power can prove extremely difficult due to the variability of emergency and, above all, trauma settings.

Acknowledgements

We thank Dr. Eleonora Ferretti, Head of the S.S. Clinical Trial Centre-Research and Statistics Infrastructure – Scientific Department, for her invaluable efforts in supporting research activities at our Institution.

Conflict of interest

The authors declare no conflict of interest.

Author details

Ruggero Bollino[1*†], Helen Yu[1†], Davide Luppi[1] and Maurizio Zizzo[2]

1 General and Emergency Surgery Unit Azienda USL–IRCCS Reggio Emilia, Reggio Emilia, Italy

2 Surgical Oncology Unit Azienda USL–IRCCS Reggio Emilia, Reggio Emilia, Italy

*Address all correspondence to: ruggerobollino@gmail.com

† These authors contributed equally.

References

[1] Wilmore DW, Kehlet H. Clinical review: Recent advances: Management of patients in fast track surgery. British Medical Journal. 2001;**322**:473-476

[2] Fearon KCH, Ljungqvist O, Von Meyenfeldt M, et al. Enhanced recovery after surgery: A consensus review of clinical care for patients undergoing colonic resection. Clinical Nutrition. 2005;**24**(3):466-477. DOI: 10.1016/j.clnu.2005.02.002

[3] Khan S, Gatt M, Horgan A, Anderson I. Guidelines for implementation of enhanced recovery protocols. In: Assoc Surg Gt Britain Irel - Issues Prof Pract. London: Association of Surgeons of Great Britain and Ireland; 2009. p. 28

[4] Gustafsson UO, Hausel J, Thorell A, Ljungqvist O, Soop M, Nygren J. Adherence to the enhanced recovery after surgery protocol and outcomes after colorectal cancer surgery. Archives of Surgery. 2011;**146**(5):571-577. DOI: 10.1001/archsurg.2010.309

[5] Gustafsson UO, Scott MJ, Hubner M, et al. Guidelines for perioperative care in elective colorectal surgery: Enhanced recovery after surgery (ERAS®) society recommendations: 2018. World Journal of Surgery. 2019;**43**(3):659-695. DOI: 10.1007/s00268-018-4844-y

[6] Ljungqvist O, Francis N, Urman R. Enhanced Recovery after Surgery: A Complete Guide to Optimizing Outcomes. Cham, Switzerland: Springer; 2020. DOI: 10.1007/978-3-030-33443-7

[7] Baron DM, Hochrieser H, Posch M, et al. Preoperative anaemia is associated with poor clinical outcome in non-cardiac surgery patients. British Journal of Anaesthesia. 2014;**113**(3):416-423. DOI: 10.1093/bja/aeu098

[8] Correia MI, Caiaffa WT, da Silva AL, Waitzberg DL. Risk factors for malnutrition in patients undergoing gastroenterological and hernia surgery: An analysis of 374 patients. Nutrición Hospitalaria. 2001;**16**(2):59-64

[9] Kang CY, Halabi WJ, Chaudhry OO, et al. Risk factors for anastomotic leakage after anterior resection for rectal cancer. Archives of Surgery. 2013;**148**(1):65-71. DOI: 10.1001/2013.jamasurg.2

[10] Simonsen C, De Heer P, Bjerre ED, et al. Sarcopenia and postoperative complication risk in gastrointestinal surgical oncology. Annals of Surgery. 2018;**268**(1):58-69. DOI: 10.1097/SLA.0000000000002679

[11] Klein S, Kinney J, Jeejeebhoy K, et al. Nutrition support in clinical practice: Review of published data and recommendations for future research directions. Summary of a conference sponsored by the National Institutes of Health, American Society for Parenteral and Enteral Nutrition, and American Society for Clinical Nutrition. The American Journal of Clinical Nutrition. 1997;**66**(3):683-706. DOI: 10.1093/ajcn/66.3.683

[12] Thomsen T, Villebro N, Møller AM. Interventions for preoperative smoking cessation. Cochrane Database of Systematic Reviews (John Wiley & Sons, Ltd). 2014;**2014**(3). SN: 1465-1858. DOI: 10.1002/14651858.CD002294.pub4

[13] Pierre S, Rivera C, Le Maître B, et al. Guidelines on smoking management during the perioperative period. Anaesthesia, Critical Care & Pain Medicine. 2017;**36**(3):195-200. DOI: 10.1016/j.accpm.2017.02.002

[14] Egholm JWM, Pedersen B, Møller AM, Adami J, Juhl CB, Tønnesen H. Perioperative alcohol cessation intervention for postoperative complications. Cochrane Database of Systematic Reviews (John Wiley & Sons, Ltd). 2018;**2018**(11). SN: 1465-1858. DOI: 10.1002/14651858.CD008343.pub3

[15] Gillis C, Buhler K, Bresee L, et al. Effects of nutritional Prehabilitation, with and without exercise, on outcomes of patients who undergo colorectal surgery: A systematic review and meta-analysis. Gastroenterology. 2018;**155**(2):391-410.e4. DOI: 10.1053/j.gastro.2018.05.012

[16] Crowe PJ, Dennison A, Royle GT. The effect of pre-operative glucose loading on postoperative nitrogen metabolism. The British Journal of Surgery. 1984;**71**(8):635-637. DOI: 10.1002/bjs.1800710828

[17] Ljungqvist O. Modulating postoperative insulin resistance by preoperative carbohydrate loading. Best Practice & Research. Clinical Anaesthesiology. 2009;**23**(4):401-409. DOI: 10.1016/j.bpa.2009.08.004

[18] Nygren JO, Thorell A, Soop M, et al. Perioperative insulin and glucose infusion maintains normal insulin sensitivity after surgery. American Journal of Physiology. Endocrinology and Metabolism. 1998;**275**(1):38-31. DOI: 10.1152/ajpendo.1998.275.1.e140

[19] Tall J, Nygren J. In: Ljungqvist O, Francis NK, Urman RD, editors. Preoperative Fasting and Carbohydrate Treatment BT - Enhanced Recovery after Surgery: A Complete Guide to Optimizing Outcomes. Cham: Springer International Publishing; 2020. pp. 31-36. DOI: 10.1007/978-3-030-33443-7_4

[20] Rockall TA, Singh R. In: Ljungqvist O, Francis NK, Urman RD, editors. Bowel Preparation: Always, Sometimes, Never? BT - Enhanced Recovery after Surgery: A Complete Guide to Optimizing Outcomes. Cham: Springer International Publishing; 2020. pp. 105-116. DOI: 10.1007/978-3-030-33443-7_12

[21] Fawcett WJ. In: Ljungqvist O, Francis NK, Urman RD, editors. Anesthetic Management and the Role of the Anesthesiologist in Reducing Surgical Stress and Improving Recovery BT - Enhanced Recovery after Surgery: A Complete Guide to Optimizing Outcomes. Cham: Springer International Publishing; 2020. pp. 131-140. DOI: 10.1007/978-3-030-33443-7_14

[22] Brandstrup B, Tønnesen H, Beier-Holgersen R, et al. Effects of intravenous fluid restriction on postoperative complications: Comparison of two perioperative fluid regimens - A randomized assessor-blinded Multicenter trial. Annals of Surgery. 2003;**238**(5):641-648. DOI: 10.1097/01.sla.0000094387.50865.23

[23] Myles PS, Bellomo R, Corcoran T, et al. Restrictive versus Liberal fluid therapy for major abdominal surgery. The New England Journal of Medicine. 2018;**378**(24):2263-2274. DOI: 10.1056/nejmoa1801601

[24] Hunter JM. Reversal of residual neuromuscular block: Complications associated with perioperative management of muscle relaxation. British Journal of Anaesthesia. 2017;**119**:i53-i62. DOI: 10.1093/bja/aex318

[25] Young-Fadok TM, Craner RC. In: Ljungqvist O, Francis NK, Urman RD, editors. Regional Anesthesia Techniques for Abdominal Operations BT - Enhanced Recovery after Surgery: A Complete Guide to Optimizing Outcomes. Cham: Springer International

Publishing; 2020. pp. 149-162. DOI: 10.1007/978-3-030-33443-7_16

[26] Watt DG, McSorley ST, Horgan PG, McMillan DC. Enhanced recovery after surgery: Which components, if any, impact on the systemic inflammatory response following colorectal surgery? A systematic review. Medicine (United States). 2015;**94**(36):1-10. DOI: 10.1097/MD.0000000000001286

[27] Kennedy RH, Francis A, Dutton S, et al. EnROL: A multicentre randomised trial of conventional versus laparoscopic surgery for colorectal cancer within an enhanced recovery programme. BMC Cancer. 2012;**12**(1):1. DOI: 10.1186/1471-2407-12-181

[28] Salvo G, Ramirez PT. In: Ljungqvist O, Francis NK, Urman RD, editors. Tubes and Drains: Current Updates on Evidence on their Role within Recovery BT - Enhanced Recovery after Surgery: A Complete Guide to Optimizing Outcomes. Cham: Springer International Publishing; 2020. pp. 185-192. DOI: 10.1007/978-3-030-33443-7_20

[29] Nelson R, Edwards S, Tse B. Prophylactic nasogastric decompression after abdominal surgery. Cochrane Database of Systematic Reviews (John Wiley & Sons, Ltd). 2004;(3). SN: 1465-1858. DOI: 10.1002/14651858.CD004929.pub2

[30] Wang D, Li T, Yu J, Hu Y, Liu H, Li G. Is nasogastric or Nasojejunal decompression necessary following gastrectomy for gastric cancer? A systematic review and meta-analysis of randomised controlled trials. Journal of Gastrointestinal Surgery. 2015;**19**(1):195-204. DOI: 10.1007/s11605-014-2648-4

[31] Weijs TJ, Kumagai K, Berkelmans GHK, Nieuwenhuijzen GAP, Nilsson M, Luyer MDP. Nasogastric decompression following esophagectomy: A systematic literature review and meta-analysis. Diseases of the Esophagus. 2017;**30**(3):1-8. DOI: 10.1111/dote.12530

[32] Lewis SJ, Andersen HK, Thomas S. Early enteral nutrition within 24 h of intestinal surgery versus later commencement of feeding: A systematic review and meta-analysis. Journal of Gastrointestinal Surgery. 2009;**13**(3):569-575. DOI: 10.1007/s11605-008-0592-x

[33] Willcutts KF, Chung MC, Erenberg CL, Finn KL, Schirmer BD, Byham-Gray LD. Early oral feeding as compared with traditional timing of oral feeding after upper gastrointestinal surgery. Annals of Surgery. 2016;**264**(1):54-63. DOI: 10.1097/SLA.0000000000001644

[34] Klek S, Kulig J, Sierzega M, et al. The impact of immunostimulating nutrition on infectious complications after upper gastrointestinal surgery: A prospective, randomized, clinical trial. Annals of Surgery. 2008;**248**(2):212-220. DOI: 10.1097/SLA.0b013e318180a3c1

[35] Moya P, Soriano-Irigaray L, Ramirez JM, et al. Perioperative standard oral nutrition supplements versus immunonutrition in patients undergoing colorectal resection in an enhanced recovery (ERAS) protocol. Medicine (United States). 2016;**95**(21):1-11. DOI: 10.1097/MD.0000000000003704

[36] Bragg D, El-Sharkawy AM, Psaltis E, Maxwell-Armstrong CA, Lobo DN. Postoperative ileus: Recent developments in pathophysiology and management. Clinical Nutrition. 2015;**34**(3):367-376. DOI: 10.1016/j.clnu.2015.01.016

[37] Adiamah A, Lobo DN. In: Ljungqvist O, Francis NK, Urman RD, editors. Postoperative Ileus: Prevention

and Treatment BT - Enhanced Recovery after Surgery: A Complete Guide to Optimizing Outcomes. Cham: Springer International Publishing; 2020. pp. 249-257. DOI: 10.1007/978-3-030-33443-7_27

[38] Han H-S, Park DJ. In: Ljungqvist O, Francis NK, Urman RD, editors. Antibiotic Prophylaxis and Surgical Site Infection Prevention BT - Enhanced Recovery after Surgery: A Complete Guide to Optimizing Outcomes. Cham: Springer International Publishing; 2020. pp. 259-267. DOI: 10.1007/978-3-030-33443-7_28

[39] Pędziwiatr M, Mavrikis J, Witowski J, et al. Current status of enhanced recovery after surgery (ERAS) protocol in gastrointestinal surgery. Medical Oncology. 2018;**35**(6):1-8. DOI: 10.1007/s12032-018-1153-0

[40] Ni X, Jia D, Chen Y, Wang L, Suo J. Is the enhanced recovery after surgery (ERAS) program effective and safe in laparoscopic colorectal cancer surgery? A meta-analysis of randomized controlled trials. Journal of Gastrointestinal Surgery. Jul 2019;**23**(7):1502-1512. DOI: 10.1007/s11605-019-04170-8. Epub 2019 Mar 11. PMID: 30859422

[41] Greco M, Capretti G, Beretta L, Gemma M, Pecorelli N, Braga M. Enhanced recovery program in colorectal surgery: A meta-analysis of randomized controlled trials. World Journal of Surgery. 2014;**38**(6):1531-1541. DOI: 10.1007/s00268-013-2416-8

[42] Passeri M, Tezber K, Eller M, Aviles C, Iannitti DA, Vrochides D. In: Ljungqvist O, Francis NK, Urman RD, editors. Readmission Challenges and Impacts within ERAS BT - Enhanced Recovery after Surgery: A Complete Guide to Optimizing Outcomes. Cham: Springer International Publishing; 2020. pp. 297-303. DOI: 10.1007/978-3-030-33443-7_32

[43] Møller MH, Adamsen S, Thomsen RW, Møller AM. Multicentre trial of a perioperative protocol to reduce mortality in patients with peptic ulcer perforation. The British Journal of Surgery. 2011;**98**(6):802-810. DOI: 10.1002/bjs.7429

[44] Huddart S, Peden CJ, Swart M, et al. Use of a pathway quality improvement care bundle to reduce mortality after emergency laparotomy. The British Journal of Surgery. 2015;**102**(1):57-66. DOI: 10.1002/bjs.9658

[45] Ebm C, Aggarwal G, Huddart S, Cecconi M, Quiney N. Cost-effectiveness of a quality improvement bundle for emergency laparotomy. BJS Open. 2018;**2**(4):262-269. DOI: 10.1002/bjs5.62

[46] Lohsiriwat V. Enhanced recovery after surgery vs conventional care in emergency colorectal surgery. World Journal of Gastroenterology. 2014;**20**(38):13950-13955. DOI: 10.3748/wjg.v20.i38.13950

[47] Gonenc M, Dural AC, Celik F, et al. Enhanced postoperative recovery pathways in emergency surgery: A randomised controlled clinical trial. American Journal of Surgery. 2014;**207**(6):807-814. DOI: 10.1016/j.amjsurg.2013.07.025

[48] Quiney N, Aggarwal G, Scott M, Dickinson M. Survival after emergency general surgery: What can we learn from enhanced recovery programmes? World Journal of Surgery. 2016;**40**(6):1283-1287. DOI: 10.1007/s00268-016-3418-0

[49] Wisely JC, Barclay KL. Effects of an enhanced recovery after surgery programme on emergency surgical patients. ANZ Journal of Surgery. 2016;**86**(11):883-888. DOI: 10.1111/ans.13465

[50] Mohsina S, Shanmugam D, Sureshkumar S, Kundra P,

Mahalakshmy T, Kate V. Adapted ERAS pathway vs. standard care in patients with perforated duodenal ulcer—A randomized controlled trial. Journal of Gastrointestinal Surgery. 2018;**22**(1):107-116. DOI: 10.1007/s11605-017-3474-2

[51] Lohsiriwat V. Enhanced recovery after surgery for emergency colorectal surgery: Are there any differences between intra-abdominal infection and other indications? Journal of Visceral Surgery. 2019;**156**(6):489-496. DOI: 10.1016/j.jviscsurg.2019.05.006

[52] Viñas X, Macarulla E, Brugiotti C, et al. Feasibility and effects of enhanced recovery vs. conventional care after emergency colon surgery for patients with left colon perforation. Scientific Reports. 2020;**10**(1):1-7. DOI: 10.1038/s41598-020-64242-7

[53] NELA Project Team. Fifth Patient Report of the National Emergency Laparotomy Audit Fifth Patient Report of the National Emergency Laparotomy Audit December 2017 to November 2018. 2019

[54] Mihai P, Ponchietti L, Casas IM, Peter Svenningsen MZ. Enhanced recovery after emergency surgery: A systematic review. Bulletin of Emergency and Trauma. 2017;**5**(2):70-78. DOI: 10.1007/s12262-021-03200-7

[55] Paduraru M, Ponchietti L, Casas IM, et al. Enhanced recovery after surgery (ERAS) - the evidence in geriatric emergency surgery: A systematic review. Chirurgia (Bucur). 2017;**112**(5):546-557. DOI: 10.21614/chirurgia.112.5.546

[56] Jovanović G, Jakovljević DK, Lukić-Šarkanović M. Enhanced recovery in surgical intensive care: A review. Frontiers in Medicine. 2018;**5**:1-6. DOI: 10.3389/fmed.2018.00256

[57] Hajibandeh S, Hajibandeh S, Bill V, Satyadas T. Meta-analysis of enhanced recovery after surgery (ERAS) protocols in emergency abdominal surgery. World Journal of Surgery. 2020;**44**(5):1336-1348. DOI: 10.1007/s00268-019-05357-5

[58] Uchino H, Nguyen-Powanda P, Tokuno J, Kouyoumdjian A, Fiore JF Jr, Grushka J. Enhanced recovery protocols in trauma and emergency abdominal surgery: A scoping review. European Journal of Trauma and Emergency Surgery. Dec 2023;**49**(6):2401-2412. DOI: 10.1007/s00068-023-02337-2. Epub 2023 Jul 28. PMID: 37505285

[59] McKechnie T, Tessier L, Archer V, Park L, Cohen D, Levac B, et al. Enhanced recovery after surgery protocols following emergency intra-abdominal surgery: A systematic review and meta-analysis. European Journal of Trauma and Emergency Surgery. 20 Nov 2023. DOI: 10.1007/s00068-023-02387-6. PMID: 37985500

[60] Mac Curtain BM, O'Mahony A, Temperley HC, Ng ZQ. Enhanced recovery after surgery protocols and emergency surgery: A systematic review and meta-analysis of randomized controlled trials. ANZ Journal of Surgery. 2023;**93**(7-8):1780-1786. DOI: 10.1111/ans.18550

[61] Peden CJ, Aggarwal G, Aitken RJ, et al. Guidelines for perioperative Care for Emergency Laparotomy Enhanced Recovery after Surgery (ERAS) society recommendations: Part 1—Preoperative: Diagnosis, rapid assessment and optimization. World Journal of Surgery. 2021;**45**(5):1272-1290. DOI: 10.1007/s00268-021-05994-9

[62] NICE. Acutely ill patients in hospital: Recognising and responding to deterioration. In: NICE; 2007. Clinical Guideline CG50. London: Natl Inst Heal Clin Excell; 2007. pp. 1-107. Available from: https://www.nice.org.uk/guidance/cg50

[63] Azuhata T, Kinoshita K, Kawano D, et al. Time from admission to initiation of surgery for source control is a critical determinant of survival in patients with gastrointestinal perforation with associated septic shock. Critical Care. 2014;**18**(3):1-10. DOI: 10.1186/cc13854

[64] Peacock O, Bassett MG, Kuryba A, et al. Thirty-day mortality in patients undergoing laparotomy for small bowel obstruction. The British Journal of Surgery. 2018;**105**(8):1006-1013. DOI: 10.1002/bjs.10812

[65] Prytherch DR, Whiteley MS, Higgins B, Weaver PC, Prout WG, Powell SJ. POSSUM and Portsmouth POSSUM for predicting mortality. The British Journal of Surgery. 1998;**85**(9):1217-1220. DOI: 10.1046/j.1365-2168.1998.00840.x

[66] Stonelake S, Thomson P, Suggett N. Identification of the high risk emergency surgical patient: Which risk prediction model should be used? Annals of Medicine and Surgery. 2015;**4**(3):240-247. DOI: 10.1016/j.amsu.2015.07.004

[67] Rhodes A, Evans LE, Alhazzani W, et al. Surviving Sepsis Campaign: International Guidelines for Management of Sepsis and Septic Shock: 2016. Vol. 43. Berlin Heidelberg: Springer; 2017. DOI: 10.1007/s00134-017-4683-6

[68] Buck DL, Vester-Andersen M, Møller MH. Surgical delay is a critical determinant of survival in perforated peptic ulcer. The British Journal of Surgery. 2013;**100**(8):1045-1049. DOI: 10.1002/bjs.9175

[69] Boyd-Carson H, Doleman B, Cromwell D, et al. Delay in source control in perforated peptic ulcer leads to 6% increased risk of death per hour: A Nationwide cohort study. World Journal of Surgery. 2020;**44**(3):869-875. DOI: 10.1007/s00268-019-05254-x

[70] Peden CJ, Aggarwal G, Aitken RJ, et al. Enhanced recovery after surgery (ERAS®) society consensus guidelines for emergency laparotomy part 3: Organizational aspects and general considerations for Management of the Emergency Laparotomy Patient. World Journal of Surgery. 2023;**47**(8):1881-1898. DOI: 10.1007/s00268-023-07039-9

[71] Galloway DA, Laimins LA, Division B, Hutchinson F. Guideline for postoperative delirium in older adults. American Geriatrics Society abstracted clinical practice. Journal of the American Geriatrics Society. 2016;**63**(1):87-92. DOI: 10.1111/jgs.13281.American

[72] Keeling D, Tait RC, Watson H. British committee of standards for haematology. Peri-operative management of anticoagulation and antiplatelet therapy. British Journal of Haematology. 2016;**175**(4):602-613. DOI: 10.1111/bjh.14344

[73] Yatabe T, Inoue S, Sakaguchi M, Egi M. The optimal target for acute glycemic control in critically ill patients: A network meta-analysis. Intensive Care Medicine. 2017;**43**(1):16-28. DOI: 10.1007/s00134-016-4558-2

[74] Stept WJ, Safar P. Rapid induction-intubation for prevention of gastric-content aspiration. Anesthesia & Analgesia. Jul-Aug 1970;**49**(4):633-636. PMID: 5534675

[75] Scott MJ, Aggarwal G, Aitken RJ, et al. Consensus guidelines for perioperative care for emergency laparotomy enhanced recovery after surgery (ERAS®) society recommendations part 2—Emergency laparotomy: Intra- and postoperative care. World Journal of Surgery. 2023;**47**(8):1850-1880. DOI: 10.1007/s00268-023-07020-6

[76] Watson X, Chereshneva M, Odor PM, et al. Adoption of lung

protective ventilation in patients undergoing emergency laparotomy: The ALPINE study. A prospective multicentre observational study. British Journal of Anaesthesia. 2018;**121**(4):909-917. DOI: 10.1016/j.bja.2018.04.048

[77] Young CC, Harris EM, Vacchiano C, et al. Lung-protective ventilation for the surgical patient: International expert panel-based consensus recommendations. British Journal of Anaesthesia. 2019;**123**(6):898-913. DOI: 10.1016/j.bja.2019.08.017

[78] Ventham NT, Hughes M, O'Neill S, Johns N, Brady RR, Wigmore SJ. Systematic review and meta-analysis of continuous local anaesthetic wound infiltration versus epidural analgesia for postoperative pain following abdominal surgery. The British Journal of Surgery. 2013;**100**(10):1280-1289. DOI: 10.1002/bjs.9204

[79] Karthikesalingam A, Walsh SR, Markar SR, Sadat U, Tang TY, Malata CM. Continuous wound infusion of local anaesthetic agents following colorectal surgery: Systematic review and meta-analysis. World Journal of Gastroenterology. 2008;**14**(34):5301-5305. DOI: 10.3748/wjg.14.5301

[80] Yu N, Long X, Lujan-Hernandez JR, Succar J, Xin X, Wang X. Transversus abdominis-plane block versus local anesthetic wound infiltration in lower abdominal surgery: A systematic review and meta-analysis of randomized controlled trials. BMC Anesthesiology. 2014;**14**(1):1-9. DOI: 10.1186/1471-2253-14-121

[81] Marks JL, Ata B, Tulandi T. Systematic review and metaanalysis of intraperitoneal instillation of local anesthetics for reduction of pain after gynecologic laparoscopy. Journal of Minimally Invasive Gynecology. 2012;**19**(5):545-553. DOI: 10.1016/j.jmig.2012.04.002

[82] Parthasarathy M, Greensmith M, Bowers D, Groot-Wassink T. Risk factors for anastomotic leakage after colorectal resection: A retrospective analysis of 17 518 patients. Colorectal Disease. 2017;**19**(3):288-298. DOI: 10.1111/codi.13476

[83] Zakrison T, Nascimento BA, Tremblay LN, Kiss A, Rizoli SB. Perioperative vasopressors are associated with an increased risk of gastrointestinal anastomotic leakage. World Journal of Surgery. 2007;**31**(8):1627-1634. DOI: 10.1007/s00268-007-9113-4

[84] Waibel BH, Rotondo MF. Damage control for intra-abdominal sepsis. The Surgical Clinics of North America. 2012;**92**(2):243-257. DOI: 10.1016/j.suc.2012.01.006

[85] van Ruler O, Boermeester MA. Surgical treatment of secondary peritonitis: A continuing problem. Der Chirurg. 2017;**88**(1):1-6. DOI: 10.1007/s00104-015-0121-x

[86] Tolonen M, Mentula P, Sallinen V, Rasilainen S, Bäcklund M, Leppäniemi A. Open abdomen with vacuum-assisted wound closure and mesh-mediated fascial traction in patients with complicated diffuse secondary peritonitis: A single-center 8-year experience. Journal of Trauma and Acute Care Surgery. 2017;**82**(6):1100-1105. DOI: 10.1097/TA.0000000000001452

[87] Di Saverio S, Podda M, De Simone B, et al. Diagnosis and treatment of acute appendicitis: 2020 update of the WSES Jerusalem guidelines. World Journal of Emergency Surgery: WJES. 2020;**15**(1):1-42. DOI: 10.1186/s13017-020-00306-3

[88] Ansari M, Akhtar A, Haleem S, Husain M, Kumar A. Is there a role of

abdominal drainage in primarily repaired perforated peptic ulcers? Journal of Experimental and Integrative Medicine. 2012;**2**(1):47. DOI: 10.5455/jeim.201111.or.015

[89] Sartelli M, Chichom-Mefire A, Labricciosa FM, et al. The management of intra-abdominal infections from a global perspective: 2017 WSES guidelines for management of intra-abdominal infections. World Journal of Emergency Surgery: WJES. 2017;**12**(1):1-34. DOI: 10.1186/s13017-017-0141-6

[90] Ademuyiwa AO, Adisa AO, Bhangu A, et al. Routine sterile glove and instrument change at the time of abdominal wound closure to prevent surgical site infection (ChEETAh): A pragmatic, cluster-randomised trial in seven low-income and middle-income countries. Lancet. 2022;**400**(10365):1767-1776. DOI: 10.1016/S0140-6736(22)01884-0

[91] Brueckmann B, Villa-Uribe JL, Bateman BT, Grosse-Sundrup M, Hess DR, Schlett CL, et al. Development and validation of a score for prediction of postoperative respiratory complications. Anesthesiology. Jun 2013;**118**(6):1276-1285. DOI: 10.1097/ALN.0b013e318293065c. PMID: 23571640

[92] Fernandez-Bustamante A, Frendl G, Sprung J, et al. Postoperative pulmonary complications, early mortality, and hospital stay following noncardiothoracic surgery. JAMA Surgery. 2017;**152**(2):157. DOI: 10.1001/jamasurg.2016.4065

[93] Leone M, Einav S, Chiumello D, et al. Noninvasive respiratory support in the hypoxaemic peri-operative/periprocedural patient: A joint ESA/ESICM guideline. Intensive Care Medicine. 2020;**46**(4):697-713. DOI: 10.1007/s00134-020-05948-0

[94] Frat JP, Coudroy R, Marjanovic N, Thille AW. High-flow nasal oxygen therapy and noninvasive ventilation in the management of acute hypoxemic respiratory failure. Annals of Translational Medicine. 2017;**5**(14):1-8. DOI: 10.21037/atm.2017.06.52

[95] Fick DM, Semla TP, Steinman M, et al. American Geriatrics Society 2019 updated AGS beers criteria® for potentially inappropriate medication use in older adults. Journal of the American Geriatrics Society. 2019;**67**(4):674-694. DOI: 10.1111/jgs.15767

[96] Hshieh TT, Yue J, Oh E, et al. Effectiveness of multicomponent nonpharmacological delirium interventions: A meta-analysis. JAMA Internal Medicine. 2015;**175**(4):512-520. DOI: 10.1001/jamainternmed.2014.7779

[97] Hughes CG, Boncyk CS, Culley DJ, et al. American society for enhanced recovery and perioperative quality initiative joint consensus statement on postoperative delirium prevention. Anesthesia and Analgesia. 2020;**130**(6):1572-1590. DOI: 10.1213/ANE.0000000000004641

[98] Murphy PB, Vogt KN, Lau BD, et al. Venous thromboembolism prevention in emergency general surgery: A review. JAMA Surgery. 2018;**153**(5):479-486. DOI: 10.1001/jamasurg.2018.0015

[99] Ross SW, Kuhlenschmidt KM, Kubasiak JC, et al. Association of the risk of a venous thromboembolic event in emergency vs elective general surgery. JAMA Surgery. 2020;**155**(6):503-511. DOI: 10.1001/jamasurg.2020.0433

[100] Meddings J, Saint S, Fowler KE, et al. The Ann Arbor criteria for appropriate urinary catheter use in hospitalized medical patients: Results obtained by using the RAND/UCLA

appropriateness method. Annals of Internal Medicine. 2015;**162**(9):S1-S34. DOI: 10.7326/M14-1304

[101] Lee Y, McKechnie T, Springer JE, Doumouras AG, Hong D, Eskicioglu C. Optimal timing of urinary catheter removal following pelvic colorectal surgery: A systematic review and meta-analysis. International Journal of Colorectal Disease. 2019;**34**(12):2011-2021. DOI: 10.1007/s00384-019-03404-0

[102] Klappenbach RF, Yazyi FJ, Alonso Quintas F, Horna ME, Alvarez Rodríguez J, Oría A. Early oral feeding versus traditional postoperative care after abdominal emergency surgery: A randomized controlled trial. World Journal of Surgery. 2013;**37**(10):2293-2299. DOI: 10.1007/s00268-013-2143-1

[103] Masood A, Viqar S, Zia N, Ghani M, usman. Early oral feeding compared with traditional postoperative care in patients undergoing emergency abdominal surgery for perforated duodenal ulcer. Cureus. 2021;**13**(1):1-11. DOI: 10.7759/cureus.12553

[104] Weimann A, Braga M, Carli F, et al. ESPEN practical guideline: Clinical nutrition in surgery. Clinical Nutrition. 2021;**40**(7):4745-4761. DOI: 10.1016/j.clnu.2021.03.031

[105] Du Y, Karvellas CJ, Baracos V, Williams DC, Khadaroo RG. Sarcopenia is a predictor of outcomes in very elderly patients undergoing emergency surgery. Surgery (United States). 2014;**156**(3):521-527. DOI: 10.1016/j.surg.2014.04.027

[106] Ceresoli M, Braga M, Zanini N, et al. Enhanced perioperative care in emergency general surgery: The WSES position paper. World Journal of Emergency Surgery : WJES. 2023;**18**(1):1-17. DOI: 10.1186/s13017-023-00519-2

[107] Ceresoli M, Biloslavo A, Bisagni P, et al. Implementing enhanced perioperative Care in Emergency General Surgery: A prospective Multicenter observational study. World Journal of Surgery. 2023;**47**(6):1339-1347. DOI: 10.1007/s00268-023-06984-9

[108] Moydien MR, Oodit R, Chowdhury S, Edu S, Nicol AJ, Navsaria PH. Enhanced recovery after surgery (ERAS) in penetrating abdominal trauma: A prospective single-center pilot study. South African Journal of Surgery. 2016;**54**(4):7-10

[109] Purushothaman V, Priyadarshini P, Bagaria D, et al. Enhanced recovery after surgery (ERAS) in patients undergoing emergency laparotomy after trauma: A prospective, randomized controlled trial. Trauma Surgery & Acute Care Open. 2021;**6**(1):6-11. DOI: 10.1136/tsaco-2021-000698